ENTER THE KETTLEBELL!

Strength Secret of The Soviet Supermen

BY PAVEL

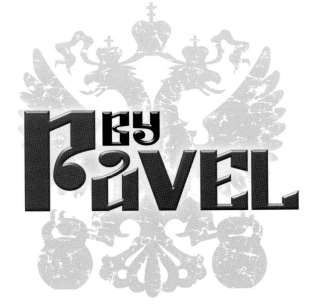

ENTER THE KETTLEBELL!

Strength Secret of The Soviet Supermen

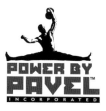

Published in the United States by:
Dragon Door Publications, Inc
5 East County Rd B, #3 • Little Canada, MN 55117
Tel: (651) 487-2180 • Fax: (651) 487-3954
Credit card orders: 1-800-899-5111
Email: support@dragondoor.com • Website: www.dragondoor.com

ISBN: 978-1-942812-13-5   1-942812-13-2

This edition first published in April 2018

Printed in China

Book design, Illustrations, logos, photo manipulation and cover by Derek Brigham
Website http//www.dbrigham.com • Tel/Fax: (763) 208-3069 • Email: bigd@dbrigham.com
Photographs by Don Pitlik: (612) 252-6797

DISCLAIMER
The author and publisher of this material are not responsible in any manner whatsoever for any injury that may occur through following the instructions contained in this material. The activities, physical and otherwise, described herein for informational purposes only, may be too strenuous or dangerous for some people and the reader(s) should consult a physician before engaging in them.

TABLE OF CONTENTS

CHAPTER 1: ENTER THE KETTLEBELL!

CHAPTER 4: A STEP-BY-STEP GUIDE TO BECOMING A MAN AMONG MEN

CHAPTER 5: FAQ

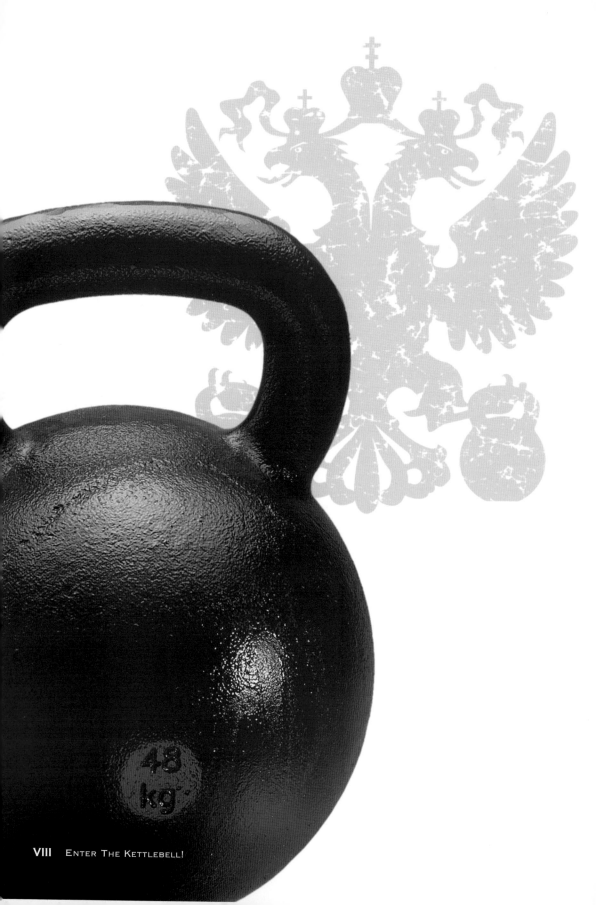

FOREWORD BY DAN JOHN

"DO THIS!"

Within minutes of meeting Pavel Tsatsouline for the first time, I was being split fore and aft and being told to tighten my hip as Pavel slapped it. I was stiff in the hip flexors and, well, Pavel was going to do his best to fix it. All I know is that I came away from our first meeting with flexible hips, a plan for lifting for the next year, and, most important, a great respect for Pavel Tsatsouline. Since meeting Pavel, I have seen literally hundreds of his posts on the Internet, read all of his books (although, to the teacher in me, "textbooks" seems more correct), and watched his library of DVDs. Whenever I review his work, one concept comes into my head: Do This!

The greatest challenge in fitness, health, life performance, and sports is walking the narrow balance beam bwetween too much variety and no variety. You know, I love Thanksgiving dinner, but not every day. One day, someone might find the perfect diet with one superfood, but I doubt many people—short of living on a desert island—would follow this diet for very long. Pavel Tsatsouline hit the mark perfectly in his book *Power to the People!*

Power to the People! had all the earmarks of a perfect program: Do This. And, "this" was deadlifts and side presses. He offered suggestions for further variation, but, honestly, one could have a successful career with just those two lifts. I have it on good authority—several drinks at a bar with these throwers—that many world-ranked track and field throwers are currently doing JUST that workout.

So, you may well ask, why do we need another kettlebell book? Where are the mad throngs of crazed health enthusiasts demanding *Enter the Kettlebell!*? You know what? They are everywhere! Early in *Enter the Kettlebell!* Pavel quotes J.M. Martin, who writes, "I was fine doing a *Power to the People!* workout because I knew exactly what to do. The book broke it down idiot proof for me and it worked. I made enormous gains. Well, now I have a kettlebell and I want to make a set-in-stone path to follow." Martin echoes what I have heard from legions of kettlebell enthusiasts: "What do I do? I've got the book/video/DVD/workshop/seminar/article...now how do I do 'what' when?"

Enter the Kettlebell!

Personally, the RKC Program Minimum was enough for me. "Here you go...DO THIS!" could be the subtitle for the first few chapters. Two exercises. Each exercise twice a week. A push and a pull (holy Power to the People!, Batman). For the majority of kettlebell users, here you go ...a plan to follow.

Personally, the RKC Program Minimum was enough for me. "Here you go . . . DO THIS!" could be the subtitle for the first few chapters. Two exercises. Each exercise twice a week. A push and a pull (holy Power to the People!, Batman). For the majority of kettlebell users, here you go . . . a plan to follow.

Pavel, however, delivers more. The chapter on the "Rite of Passage" gives us a step-by-step approach to literally climbing the ladder of kettlebell exercises. Moreover, the section "The Hazards of Variety and How to Dodge Them" is a century of knowledge compressed into a few pages. If you liked the "old school" approach, open your eyes and see the classic training methods from a kettlebell perspective.

Clearly, this book is not the end point. Pavel notes, "I never stop polishing my training system, which is why you will find some inconsistencies between *The Russian Kettlebell Challenge* and *Enter the Kettlebell!* The latter book takes precedence. At the RKC, we never rest."

I have some simple advice for you:

Do this.

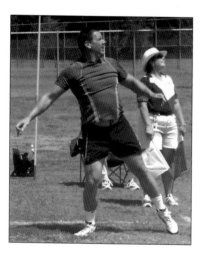

Dan John is your typical coach. A Fulbright Scholar to Egypt, Dan has advanced degrees in history and religious education. He has traveled the world dealing with parasites, customs officials and a terrible accent in every language he has learned... so much so, that both Turkish and Hebrew speakers have asked him to stop speaking their language.

When not working as a professor of religious studies, Dan is a full-time strength coach and Head Track and Field coach at Juan Diego Catholic High School in Draper, Utah. Dan has multiple national and state championships in the discus, Olympic lifting, Highland Games and the Weight Pentathlon.

Dan John is the author of two instructional DVDs, **Carried Away,** on carrying, dragging and pulling objects for strength and conditioning, and **From the Ground Up,** that teaches weightlifting fundamentals quickly and correctly, the old-school way. Both DVDs are available at www.crossfitnorcal.com/catalog/index.php. Dan also maintains the "world's largest" free website dedicated to lifting and throwing stuff at www.danjohn.org/coach.

A Step to the Left and I Shoot

Remember Robin Williams' Soviet defector character in Moscow on the Hudson? The recovering Commie just wanted to buy some coffee. In the USSR he had had two choices: 'We have coffee' or, more likely, "We are out of coffee." When he saw the variety of products in the coffee isle of a New York City supermarket, he nearly had a nervous breakdown.

The mind-boggling diversity of kettlebell exercises and applications can make the aspiring kettlebeller feel like the Russkie defector. The freestyle training program in my book *The Russian Kettlebell Challenge* kicked off a tyranny of kettlebell choices that has continued with the smorgasbord of exercises on my DVDs and those made by my senior instructors.

"Maybe someone can help," asked Comrade J.M. Martin in a thread titled "Kettlebell Confused" on our forum. "I have read all I can find on kettlebells and have to say I am at loss as to making a program. I was fine doing a *Power to the People!* workout because I knew exactly what to do. The book broke it down idiot proof for me and it worked. I made enormous gains. Well now I have a kettlebell and I want to make a set in stone path to follow...."

Enter the Kettlebell! is your "set in stone path," the ruthlessly efficient *Power to the People!* for kettlebells. A step to the left and I shoot.

Russian kettlebell power to you!

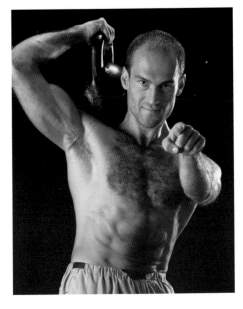

Pavel

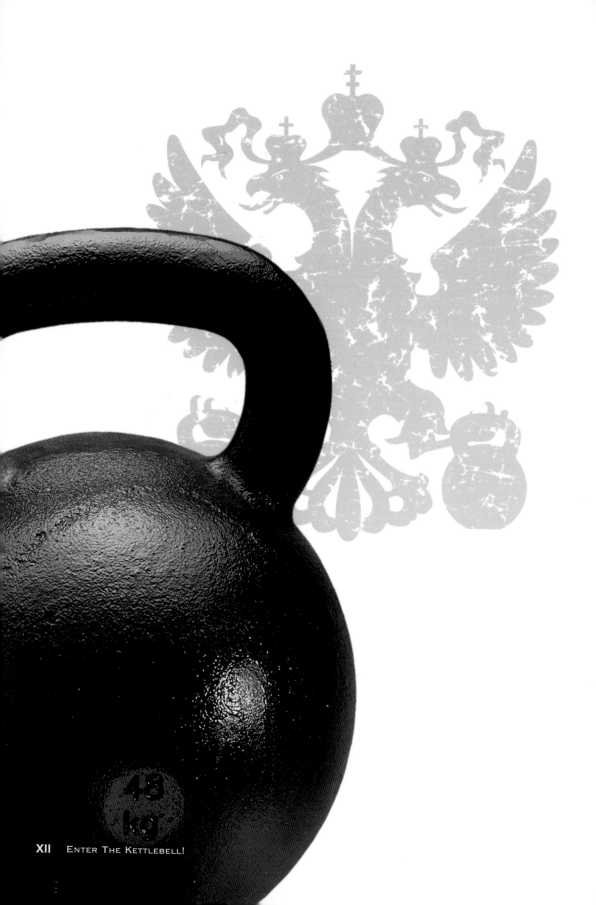

INTRODUCTION

When We Say "Strength," We Mean "Kettlebell." When We Say "Kettlebell," We Mean "Strength."

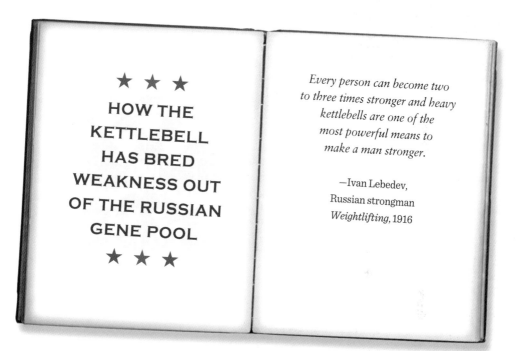

★ ★ ★

HOW THE KETTLEBELL HAS BRED WEAKNESS OUT OF THE RUSSIAN GENE POOL

★ ★ ★

Every person can become two to three times stronger and heavy kettlebells are one of the most powerful means to make a man stronger.

—Ivan Lebedev,
Russian strongman
Weightlifting, 1916

If Charles Atlas were Russian, he could have told a different story...

Sergey Mishin was a heavy, slow, decidedly nonathletic kid. He picked up his first kettlebell, a 53-pounder, at 17 and was dismayed when he could not lift it with either arm. Undeterred by his weakness, Mishin found a plumbing pipe, hammered its middle flat so it would hold the kettlebell handle in place, and started jerking the kettlebell with two hands, like a barbell. The year was 1975. Two years later, Mishin could press a 70-pounder, which he had found abandoned in a park after a festival held on Railroad Worker Day, 30 times with each arm.

Mishin kept kettlebelling in the army, and when he was discharged he bragged to a friend that he would make a Master of Sports national ranking in the first kettlebell lifting competition he entered. And he did!

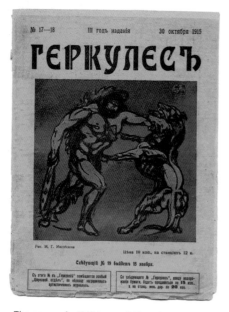

The cover of a 1915 issue of **Hercules**, Tsarist Russia's strength magazine.

Sergey lost more than 100 pounds; became fast, wiry. And went on to become the number-one kettlebell lifter in the world—170 jerks with a pair of 70-pound kettlebells in 10 minutes!—and Russia's sport legend. The president of Russia awarded Mishin a medal "For Accomplishments for the Benefit of the Motherland." (II degree).

In Russia kettlebells are a matter of national pride and a symbol of strength. In the olden days, any strongman or weightlifter was referred to as a *girevik*, or "kettlebell man." Steeled by their kettlebells, generation after generation of Russian boys has turned to men. A century before Mishin, another young boy, Pyotr Kryloff, found kettlebells at a butcher's shop. It was love at first sight. Pyotr never parted with his kettlebells, and when he became a merchant marine he took them with him around the world. Eventually the kettlebell fanatic became a circus strongman and performed until he was 60. The public called him the "King of Kettlebells." Kryloff could cross himself in the Russian Orthodox manner with a 70-pound kettlebell, military pressed the same kettlebell with one arm 88 times, and juggled *three* of them at once! Pyotr applied his kettlebell power to all sorts of feats. He broke stones with his fist, bent coins, made "ties" and "bracelets" out of strips of iron, broke horseshoes, jerked a "barbell" with two beefy soldiers sitting inside two hollow spheres, and set a few world weightlifting records.

Pyotr Kryloff, "the King of Kettlebells," could cross himself in the Russian Orthodox manner with a 70-pound kettlebell, military pressed the same kettlebell with one arm 88 times, and juggled three of them at once!

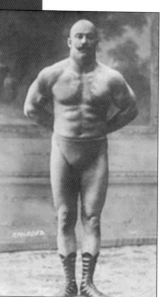

Enter "Heavy Athletics"

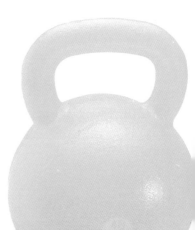

Enter "Heavy Athletics"

"It can be said with a good deal of certainty that Russian weight-lifting was born and grew thanks to the devotees of the kettlebell sport," stated Weightlifting Masters World Champion Prof. L. Dvorkin. Indeed, it was the father of kettlebells, Dr. Vladislav Krayevskiy, who coined the term "heavy athletics" (*tyazholaya atletika*), the name for the sport of Olympic weightlifting in today's Russia.

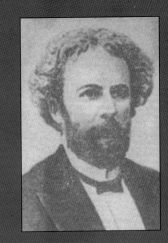

Dr. Krayevskiy, the father of kettlebells.

The Red Army and the kettlebell are inseparable. Every Russian military unit has a gym called "the courage corner." Every courage corner is equipped with kettlebells. While other countries waste time testing their troopers with push-ups, Russia tests repetition kettlebell snatches with a 53-pound kettlebell. "The rank and file of the Red Army was magnificent from a physical point of view," marveled Lt. Gen. Giffard Martel, chief of the British military mission to the USSR during World War II. "Much of the equipment we carry on vehicles accompanying the infantry is carried on the man's back in Russia. The Russians seem capable of carrying these great loads. They are exceptionally tough."

Law enforcement tactical teams—even the Russian federal tax police, who are handier with firearms than with calculators—also make kettlebells their strength training tool of choice. In the last days of the Soviet empire, the prison system was plagued with riots and hostage situations. Interior ministry troops were called in to suppress the riots. They did the job, but finesse was sure lacking. For instance, in 1986 they stormed a prison camp and burned it to the ground in the process of ruthlessly suppressing the riot.

In 1991 the interior ministry formed special tactical teams for every administrative prison district. Their mission: hostage rescue, riot suppression, search and arrest of escaped criminals. Since that memorable year when the USSR fell apart, these TAC teams have earned their keep on many occasions, in harsh Russian prisons and in Chechnya.

Russian federal prison SWAT teams are manned with former military special operators, paras, and vets of other elite services; each one had to compete against nine or more rival applicants to make the team. The selection process is similar to that of the army Spetsnaz. Here is what the trooper has to do back-to-back: a 10K forced march in full kit, an obstacle course and rappelling, plus another 10K run. A cherry on the top when you are beyond smoked is a 12-minute full-contact sparring session—with fresh opponents rotating in every three minutes. Once on the team, operators aggressively compete against their colleagues in the frequently held law enforcement sports events. Their specialties: hand-to-hand combat and the kettlebell sport. A matter of specificity and pride.

It is hard to understand the logic of governments—both Russian and American—that encourage inmates to strength train, but Russian prisoners lift kettlebells as well. You may have seen the black-and-white archive footage in a History Channel documentary about Russian organized crime—a wiry prisoner doing kettlebell swings, flips, and side presses. Some Russian prisons even host kettlebell competitions for the inmates! Go figure. Perhaps the law enforcement likes a challenge.

Why Soviet Scientists Gave the Kettlebell Two Thumbs-Up

In the 20th century, Soviet science validated what Russian hard men had known for centuries: kettlebell lifting is one of the best tools for all-around physical development.

Voropayev (1983) observ-ed two groups of college students over a period of a few years. To gauge their performance, he used a standard battery of the armed forces physical training (PT) tests: pull-ups, a standing broad jump, a 100-meter sprint, and a 1K run. The control group followed the typical university PT program, which was military oriented and emphasized the above exercises. The experimental group just lifted kettlebells. In spite of the lack of practice on the tested drills, the kettlebell group showed better scores in every one of them!

Vinogradov and Lukyanov (1986) found a very high correlation between the results posted in a kettlebell lifting competition and in a great range of dissimilar tests: strength, measured with the three powerlifts and grip strength; strength endurance, mea-sured with pull-ups and parallel bar dips; general endurance, determined by a 1K run; and work capacity and balance, measured with special tests.

Lopatin (2000) found a positive correlation between soldiers' kettlebell sport ranking and their obstacle course performance.

Kettlebells improve coordination and agility (Luchkin, 1947; Laputin, 1973).

Kettlebells develop professional applied qualities and general physical preparedness (Zikov, 1986; Griban, 1990).

Kettlebells are highly effective for building strength.

The official Soviet armed forces strength training manual approved by the ministry of defense (Burkov & Nikityuk, 1985) declared kettlebell training to be "one of the most effective means of strength development," representing "a new era in the development of human strength-potential."

Kettlebell lifting is great for your heart.

Siberian scientist Shevtsova (1993) verified what is obvious to any girevik. She studied 75 gireviks with three to five years of experience and recorded a long-term decrease in the heart rate and the blood pressure. The kettlebellers had what Russians call "a cosmonaut's blood pressure": 110/70 in the summer and 114/74 in the winter. They clocked an average resting heart rate of 56 beats per minute. The heart rate took a dive not just at rest, but also during and after exercise. And the time it took the heart to slow down back to normal, after exercise, also decreased. Besides, the experienced gireviks' systems had also adapted to be better "primed" and ready for upcoming action.

Properly used, kettlebells are surprisingly safe.

Only 8.8 percent of top Russian gireviks, members of the Russian National Team and regional teams, reported injuries in training or competition (Voropayev, 1997). A remarkably low number, especially if you consider that these are elite athletes who push their bodies over the edge.

Kettlebell training improves body composition.

According to Voropayev (1997), who studied top Russian kettlebell lifters, 21.2 percent increased their bodyweight since taking up kettlebelling, and 21.2 percent (the exact same percentage, not a typo), mostly heavyweights, decreased it. Another study of elite gireviks revealed a consistently low body fat (Gomonov, 1998).

"A girevik is characterized by a balanced development of all organs and musculature with significant hypertrophy of the muscles of the shoulder girdle." (Rasskazov, 1993).

"A girevik (legendary strongman Eugene Sandow pictured) is characterized by a balanced development of all organs and musculature with significant hypertrophy of the muscles of the shoulder girdle."—(Rasskazov, 1993)

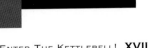

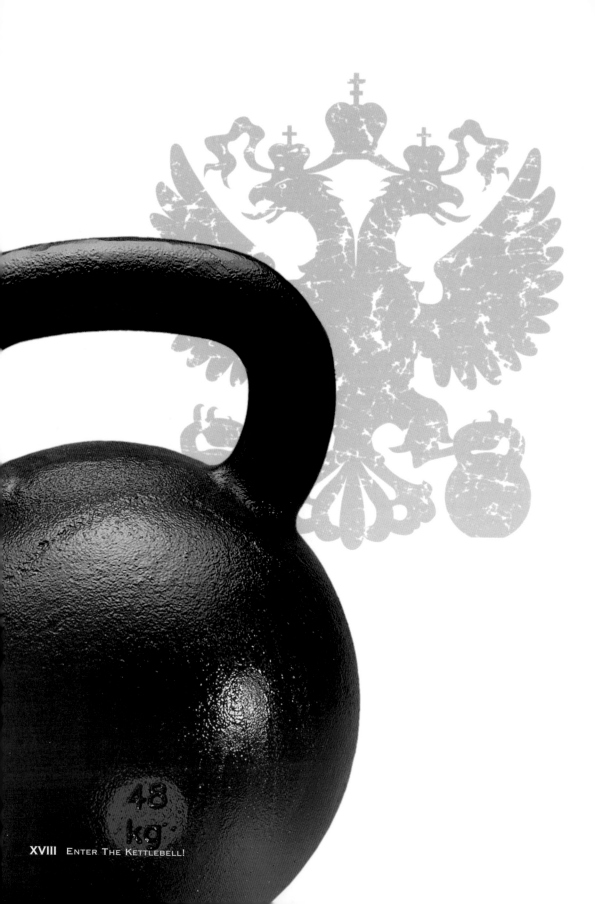

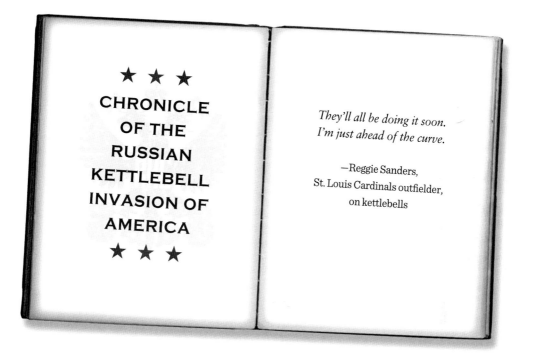

★ ★ ★ CHRONICLE OF THE RUSSIAN KETTLEBELL INVASION OF AMERICA ★ ★ ★

*They'll all be doing it soon.
I'm just ahead of the curve.*

—Reggie Sanders,
St. Louis Cardinals outfielder,
on kettlebells

American iron men of old knew the value of kettlebells. You can see a pair in the training "dungeon" of one of the greatest deadlifters of all time, Tennessee farmer Bob Peoples, who pulled more than 700 pounds weighing a buck eighty before steroids and supportive gear. Sig Klein was a big proponent of kettlebells. I bought a pair of antique 1917 American kettlebells (they look like miniature Weber grills) from a 70-year-old friend, a "once a lifter, always a lifter" who still does good mornings with 405 pounds.

Then America got prosperous and forgot its rugged frontier past. Kettlebells went the way of the California gold prospectors and the gunslingers of the Old West. The kettlebell would have remained but a chapter in manly American history if not for my friend Marty Gallagher, former Coach, Powerlifting Team USA.

Marty and I were enjoying steaks in his backyard in an undisclosed location on the East Coast. We were trading old war stories over a mouthful of Mennonite-raised beef. Marty told me about Ed Coan, Kirk Karwoski, and other champions he had coached. I told him about kettlebells.

Gallagher thoughtfully finished chewing his steak and suggested, "Why don't you write an article for *MILO*?" You know, the magazine for crazy guys who bend nails and lift rocks.

I said, "Marty, you don't get it, this is the most painful workout you could imagine, who would want to do it or even read about it?" Earlier I had made the mistake of explaining a Russian slur, the "collective farmer," to Marty. He used it on me and told me that I did not understand Americans.

The subversive *Vodka, Pickle Juice, Kettlebell Lifting, and Other Russian Pastimes* was published in 1998. The article was extremely well received by the most ruthless critics in the strength world. I started getting mail from guys with busted noses, cauliflower ears, scars, or at least Hells Angels tattoos. Incredulous, I told my friend and editor John Du Cane about it. He thought for a minute and said: "Let's do it! I'll make kettlebells and you teach people how to use them."

Behind John's reticent Cambridge demeanor is the heart of an American pioneer. A Brit who grew up in Africa, John drove from England to India—through Pakistan and Afghanistan—and lived for a few years in a Yoga community. He built his publishing company in the U.S. while driving a limousine to make ends meet. Fledgling Dragon Door Publications demanded undivided attention and John could not afford "wasting" his time on sleep. Du Cane took naps in the limo while waiting for his customers and used every spare minute to build his American Dream.

When presented with a new opportunity this rugged, self-reliant individual risked everything he had accomplished in his hard years as an entrepreneur publisher and decided to invest in manufacturing and promoting Russian kettlebells. Hindsight is always 20/20 and today it is obvious to anyone that the kettlebell is a winner. But that was not the case back then. "A cannon ball with a handle? Are you out of your mind?!"

2001 was the year of the kettlebell. Dragon Door published *The Russian Kettlebell Challenge* and forged the first US made Russian style cast iron kettlebell. RKC, the first kettlebell instructor course on American soil, also kicked off in 2001. Given the kettlebell's harsh reputation, most of my early students looked like they came from the federal witness protection program. People often ask if Steve Maxwell and I are brothers. Steve, I love you, man, but I don't think it's a compliment for either of us.

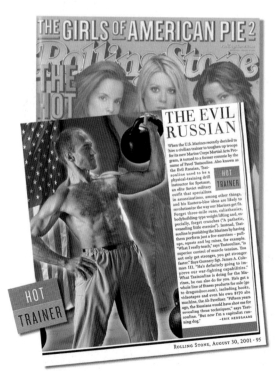

ROLLING STONE, AUGUST 30, 2001 · 95

Times change. Hard living Comrades remain the loyal core of 'the Party'. But now they have to begrudgingly share the Russian kettlebell with Hollywood movie stars and other unlikely kettlebellers. Fed up with the sissified mainstream fitness advice, smart folks go hardcore. In 2002 our Russian kettlebell made it into the *Rolling Stone's* exclusive Hot List as 'the Hot Weight'. In 2004 Dr. Randall Strossen, one of the most respected names in the strength world, stated, "In our eyes, Pavel Tsatsouline will always reign as the modern king of kettlebells since it was he who popularized them to the point where you could almost found a country filled with his converts..."

ENTER THE KETTLEBELL!

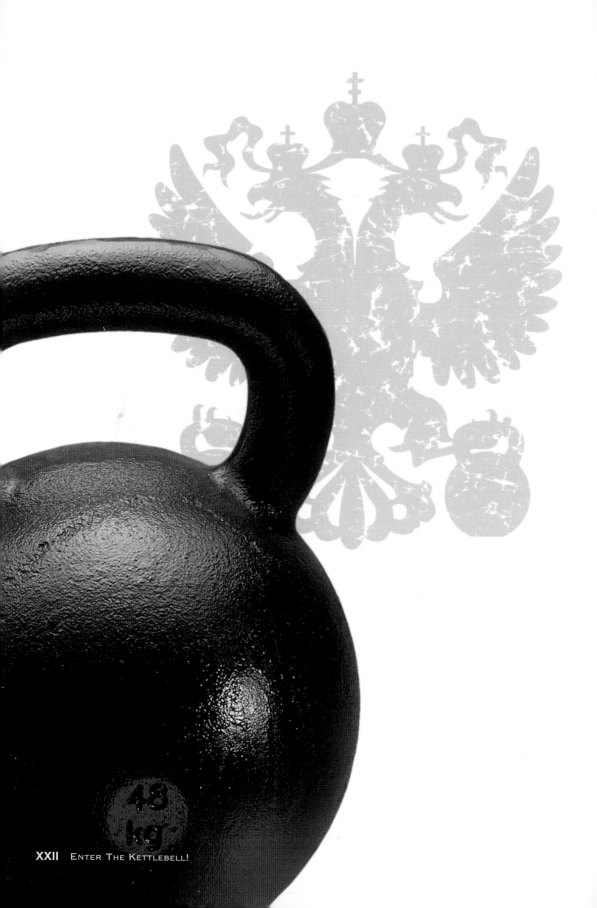

CHAPTER 1:

Enter the Kettlebell!

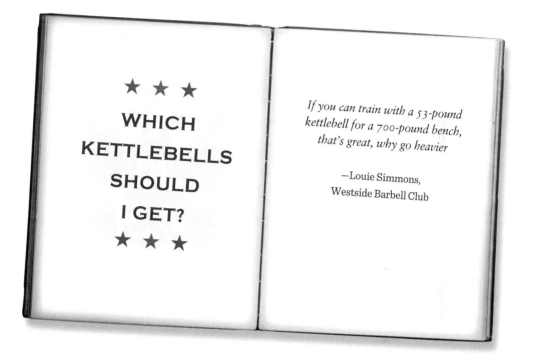

★ ★ ★

WHICH KETTLEBELLS SHOULD I GET?

★ ★ ★

If you can train with a 53-pound kettlebell for a 700-pound bench, that's great, why go heavier

—Louie Simmons,
Westside Barbell Club

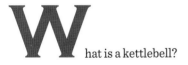hat is a kettlebell?

It's a cannonball with a handle. It's an extreme handheld gym. It's a statement: "I'm sick of your metrosexual gyms! I'm a man, and I'll train like a man!" Lifting a kettlebell is liberating and as aggressive as medieval swordplay. It's a manifestation of what Ori Hofmekler has called the "warrior instinct."

Guys name their kettlebells like they name their guns. They paint them with their units' coats of arms. They get tattoos of kettlebells. The Russian kettlebell is the Harley-Davidson of weights.

The kettlebell delivers extreme all-around fitness. All-purpose strength. Staying power. Flexibility. Fat loss without the dishonor of aerobics. All accomplished in one to two hours of weekly training. All done with one compact and virtually indestructible tool that can be used anywhere.

Russian kettlebells traditionally come in poods. One pood, an old Russian unit of measurement, equals 16 kilograms, approximately 35 pounds. The most popular sizes in Russia are 1 pood, the right kettlebell for a typical male beginner; 1 1/2 pood, or a 53-pounder, the standard issue in the military; and the "double," as the 2-pood, or 70-pound kettlebell, is called. Doubles are for advanced gireviks.

Heavy kettlebells are traditionally called "bulldogs." "Heavy" is in the eye of the beholder; we usually dump the bells heavier than 32 kilograms in that category. 48 kilograms is as heavy as traditional kettlebells go, but it does not stop Russia's strongest from going heavier. Weightlifting legend Yuri Vlasov was heartbroken when someone stole his custom-made 56-kilogram kettlebells.

Poods and Kilograms to Pounds
Approximate Conversion

Poods	kgs.	lbs.	
0.25	4	9	
0.375	6	13	The most popular sizes in Russia are shaded in red.
0.5	8	18	
0.75	12	26	
1	16	35	Male beginner's weight
1.25	20	44	
1.5	24	53	Most popular in the military
1.75	28	62	
2	32	70	Advanced men
2.5	40	88	
3	48	106	

Dragon Door makes top-quality, classic, Russian-style cast-iron kettlebells ranging from 26 to 106 pounds and rubber-coated ladies' kettlebells ranging from 9 to 18 pounds. Which ones do you need?

Start with one kettlebell; the table on the next page will help you pick the right one. If you have the funds, get a set of three or four kettlebells, referring to the table for sizes.

Do you need two kettlebells of the same size? —Not yet. Double kettlebell drills are great—look what they have done for Senior RKC Mike Mahler—but they are not for beginners. Get good with one bell, address your strength imbalances, work up to the snatch and press goals listed toward the end of this book, then we'll talk.

An average man should start with a 35-pounder. What is "average"? —Given the bench press as a typical, albeit misguided, standard of strength, men with a bench press under 200 pounds should start with a 35-pounder. If you bench more than 200, a 44 that weighs as much as a big barbell plate will do the trick. Unless you are a powerlifter or a strongman, you have no business starting with a 53.

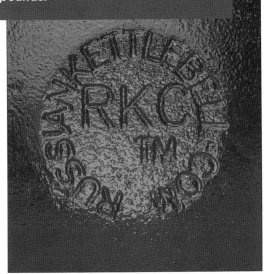

Dragon Door makes top-quality, classic, Russian-style cast-iron kettlebells ranging from 26 to 106 pounds and rubber-coated ladies' kettlebells ranging from 9 to 18 pounds.

I know, it does not sound like a lot, but a kettlebell feels a lot heavier than its weight suggests! To give you an idea, for a few years we ran an 88-pound kettlebell military press challenge at our booth at the Arnold Fitness Expo. The rules are simple: the fist must be lower than the chin at the start of the press, and the knees must remain locked. You don't even have to clean the bell because I do not want any of the "this is all technique" whining. We'll hand it to you if you insist.

Let us face it, one-arm pressing 88 pounds overhead is not a feat of strength. Definitely not for a 250-pound man who can bench close to 400 pounds. Yet most can't do it. Let this be a lesson: err on the lighter side when ordering your kettlebells. There is no dishonor. Even superpowerful men like 1,000-pound squatters RKCs Donnie Thompson and Marc Bartley find plenty of things to do with 35- and 53-pounders.

An average woman should start with an 18-pounder. A strong woman can go for a 26-pounder. Most women should advance to a 35-pounder. A few hard women will go beyond. Catherine "Steel Kate" Imes, RKC, can press the 70-pounder for a few reps, putting many men to shame.

An average woman should start with an 18-pounder. A strong woman can go for a 26-pounder. Most women should advance to a 35-pounder. A few hard women will go beyond. Catherine "Steel Kate" Imes, RKC, can press the 70-pounder for a few reps, putting many men to shame.

Start out with the Right Kettlebell!

Is It You?	Kettlebell to Start with	Ideally, Buy This Set
An average lady	18 lbs.	18, 26, 35 lbs.
A strong lady	26 lbs.	26, 35, 44 lbs.
An average gentleman	35 lbs.	35, 44, 53, 70 lbs.
A stronger-than-average gentleman	44 lbs.	44, 53, 70 lbs.
A very strong gentleman	53 lbs.	53, 70, 88 lbs.

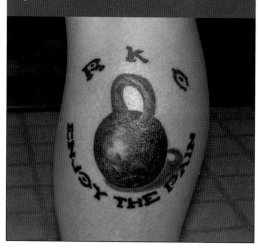

Dragon Door makes top-quality, classic, Russian-style cast-iron kettlebells ranging from 26 to 106 pounds and rubber-coated ladies' kettlebells ranging from 9 to 18 pounds.

You must have noticed that, unlike dumbbells, kettlebell weights do not go up in small increments. There is simply no need for extra iron. Inventive gireviks don't need a ton of weight to provide progressive resistance. And you get to save money and space.

Don't chase ever heavier kettlebells just for the heck of it; keep your goals in mind. Anatoly Taras, a special operations veteran and a leading hand-to-hand combat expert in the countries of the former Soviet Union, believes that once a fighting man can do 50 snatches per arm, switching hands only once, with a 24-kilogram kettlebell, he has reached the point of diminishing returns. "People of a certain personality type will ask, why not [really crank up those numbers]?" says Taras. "You could if you have the time and the desire, but it is not necessary unless your goal is setting records. Having set a few records of this kind will not make you fight any better."

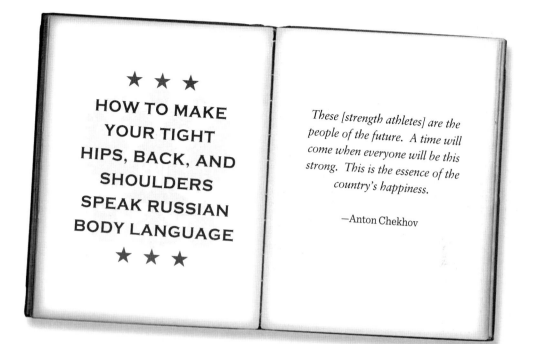

Russians are easy to spot, even if you dress them like Buckingham Palace guards. They are "the white people who look seriously ticked off," as Army Ranger vet Ellis Jones, RKC, has put it on our forum.

Then there is the walk. My wife, Julie, who has the dubious privilege of being around a lot of Russians, has pointed out the striking difference in the ways Americans and Russians walk. The former fall forward and catch themselves with their feet. The latter lead proudly with their stomachs, whether they have them or not.

For whatever cultural reasons, Americans have tight hip flexors and Russians don't. When these muscles on the top of your thighs tighten up, they make your butt stick out or, at the very least, disable you from driving your hips all the way through in a powerful pull, throw, kick, punch, or jump. Tight hip flexors act like brakes that zap your strength.

This chapter is your "kettlebell preschool." I will test and fix your lack of flexibility. Pick up your kettlebell, and we will see where you are at.

Take a comfortable stance—slightly wider than your shoulders, your feet slightly turned out—over your shiny new kettlebell. Sit back as you would in a high chair, and pick up the kettlebell with both hands by extending your hips and knees. Have someone watch you and mark off the following checklist. Don't use a mirror!

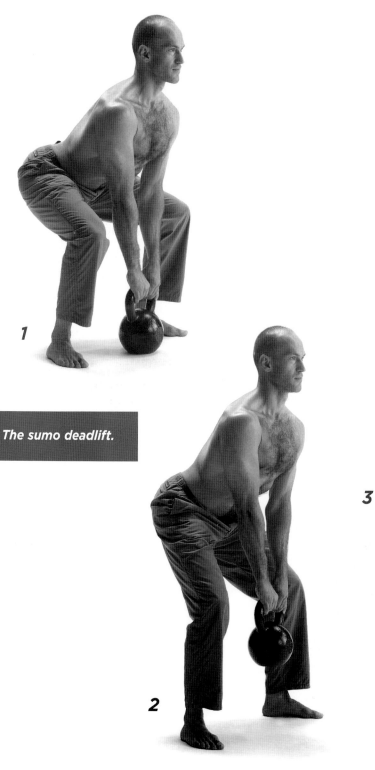

1

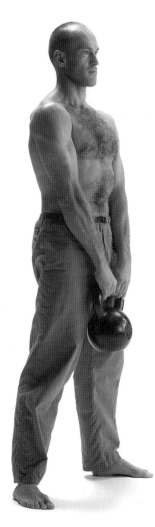

The sumo deadlift.

2

3

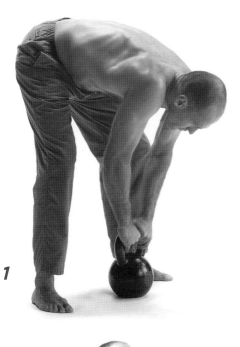

1

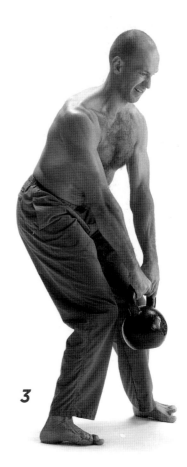

3

2

The Kettlebell Sumo Deadlift Checklist

★ Your arms are straight; the legs are doing all the lifting.

★ Your knees are pointing in the same direction as your slightly turned-out feet.

★ Your heels are planted. You are sitting back, rather than dipping down or bending forward.

★ Your back stays straight throughout. Don't confuse "straight" with "vertical"! "Straight" in this context means "not rounded."

★ You are looking straight ahead, not up or down, at all times.

If you failed any of the above requirements, you need to practice the following drill daily until you pass. No kettlebells until then, Comrade.

THE FACE-THE-WALL SQUAT

One of the exercises in John Du Cane's excellent program *The Qigong Recharge* caught my attention: the Chinese wall squat. Modified for our needs, it is an outstanding drill for developing the back and hip flexibility needed for pulling and squatting.

Stand a couple of inches away from a wall, facing it, your feet a little wider than your shoulders and slightly turned out, your arms hanging free. Keeping your feet planted—the inside edges may not come up!—and without "frogging" your knees outward, squat down as low as you can.

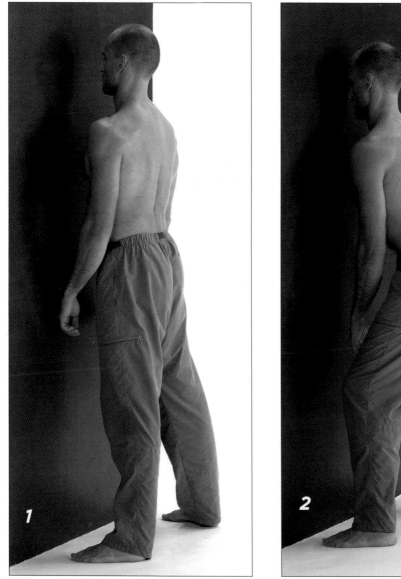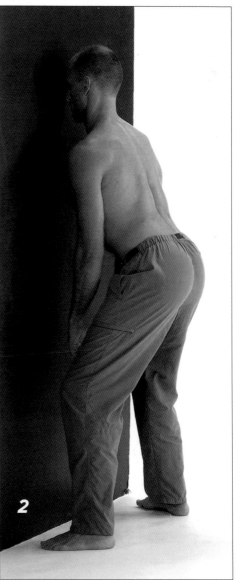

You will notice that you cannot get past a certain point without pushing your chest out and arching your lower back. And if you insist on proving me wrong and mindlessly go down, you will quickly learn that not only will you fail to descend lower than a couple of inches, your forehead or your knees will hit the wall and make you fall back. An Inspecteur Clouseau moment, yes, yes.

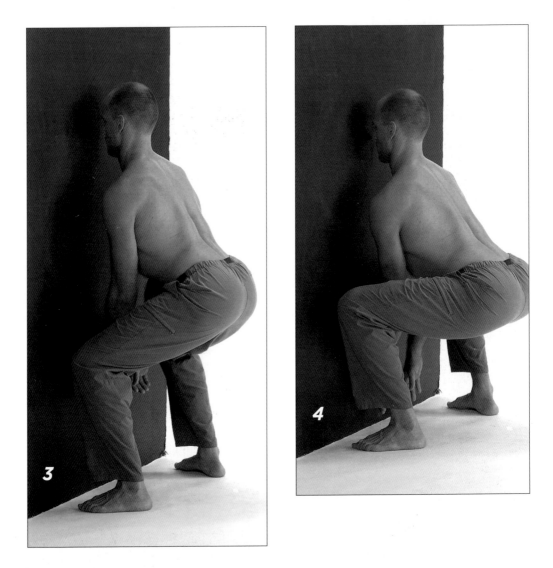

Move slowly and deliberately; use your strength. When you get tired, either in your legs or in your back, stop, shake the tension off, and come back for more when you are rested. You will make the fastest gains if you do a few reps here and there throughout the day, every day.

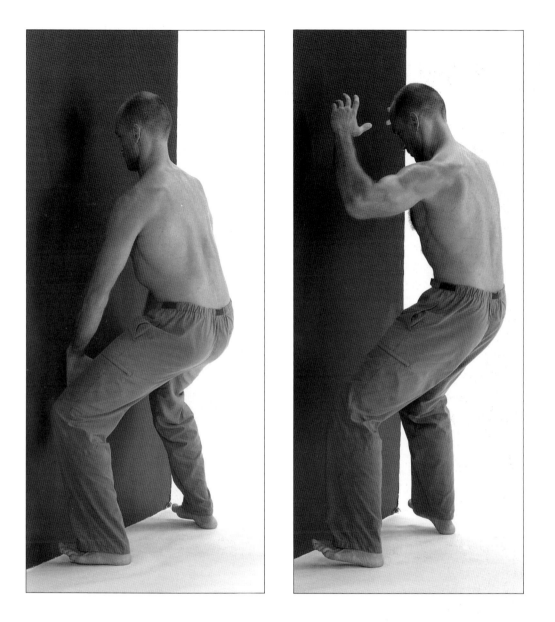

This is what happens when you don't read the instructions.

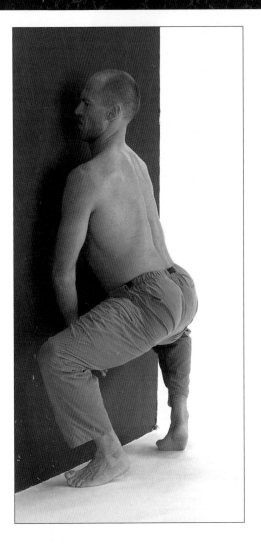

Keep working your way down into a half squat. Once you have, step a hair closer to the wall and go back to work. **The goal is to reach the point where you can squat low enough to pick up your kettlebell with your toes touching the wall.**

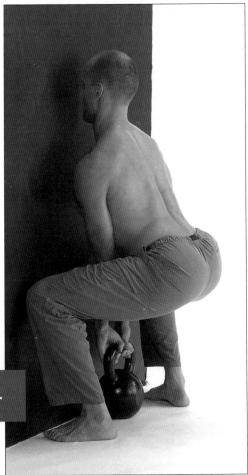

This is your face-the-wall squat goal, Comrade.

THE HALO

A great move from mobility master Steve Maxwell, Senior RKC, the halo will loosen up your shoulders. Hold a kettlebell upside down by its horns and slowly move it around your head. Work up to progressively tighter circles. Keep your glutes tight—"pinch a coin"—to protect your back.

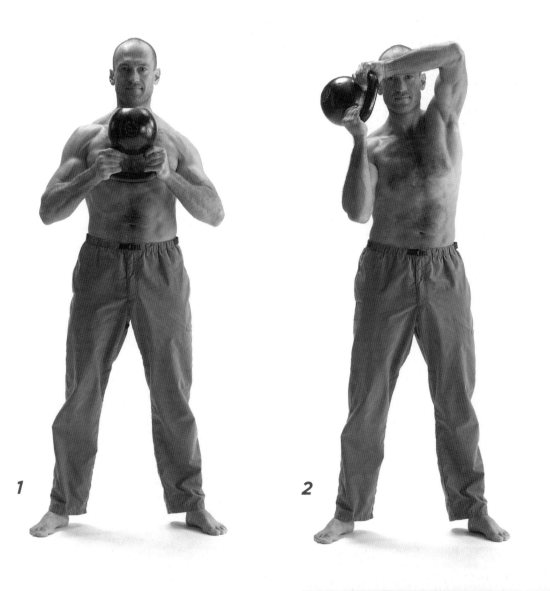

1

2

The halo.

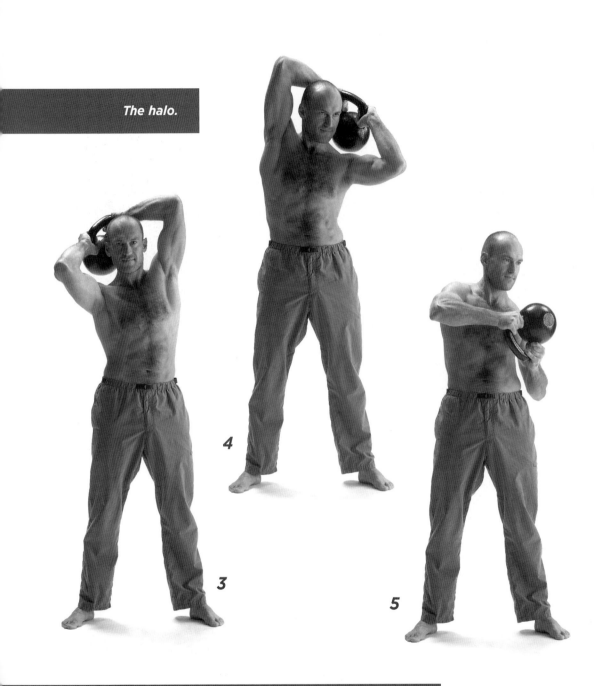

3

4

5

Keep your glutes tight—"pinch a coin"—to protect your back.

THE PUMP STRETCH

Test the top of your deadlift to find out how tight your hip flexors are.

The Kettlebell Sumo Deadlift Lockout Checklist

★ Your knees may not rebend at the top and your body may not "scoop." The movement is crisp; there is nothing flowing or touchy-feely about it!

★ On the very top, your body forms a straight line, neither your head, nor your butt, nor your knees stick out.

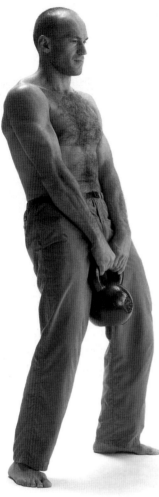

I know you have failed. Here is a drill to fix you. Practice it throughout the day, every day.

Assume a hips-high push-up position, your hands shoulder-width apart and your feet a little wider. Don't let your feet buckle in.

Keeping your elbows locked, shift your weight forward and drop your hips. Scoop up until your arms are straight and bear most of your weight. "Lengthen" your spine and look up.

Tense your glutes and push your hips forward as far as you can.

Now shift your hips side to side and turn them a few times. Try to loosen up the muscles on the top of your thighs. "Pry."

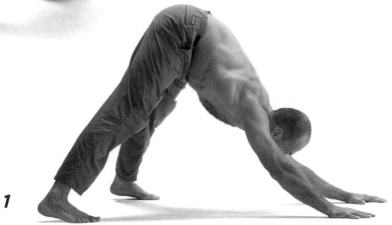

1

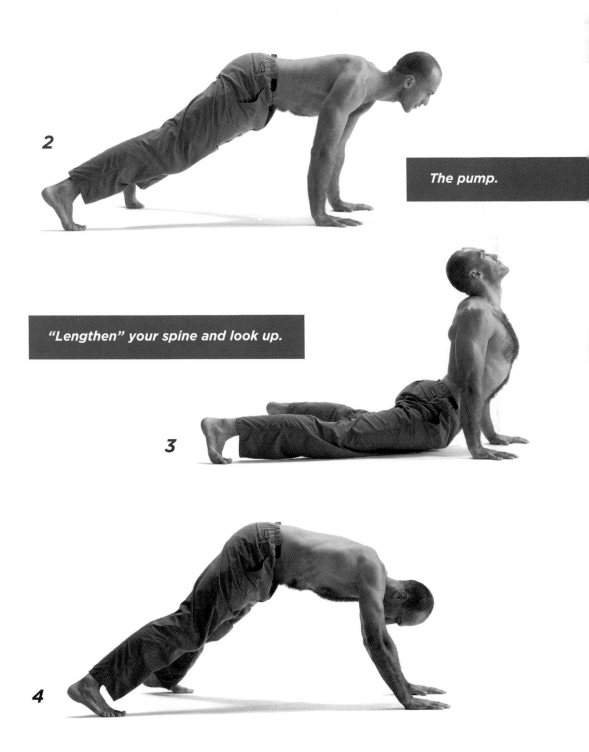

2

The pump.

"Lengthen" your spine and look up.

3

4

Now shift your hips side to side and turn them a few times. Try to loosen up the muscles on the top of your thighs. "Pry."

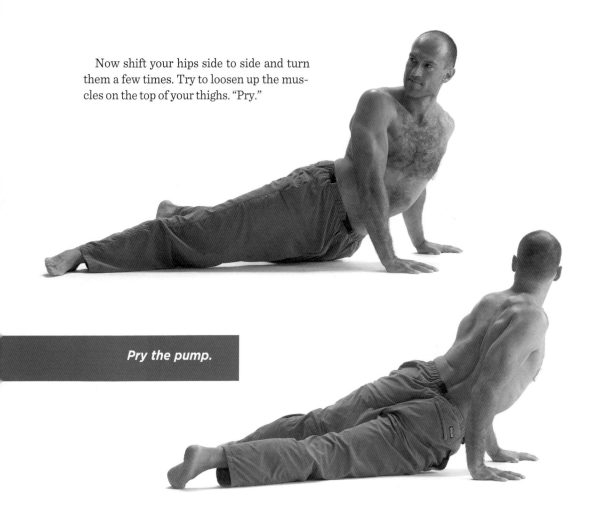

Pry the pump.

The next move will help you stretch your shoulders, another essential for kettlebell lifting.

Keeping your elbows locked, push yourself back into the starting position.

Push your hips as far back as possible and bring your chest as low to the deck as you can. Don't let your feet buckle.

Make a couple of short, springy movements, trying to bring your chest lower. A responsible training partner may push you between your shoulder blades. Note that your elbows must be completely locked at this point; otherwise you could hurt your shoulders.

And go forward again. Control the movement; focus on increasing the range of motion in your ankles, hips, back, and shoulders, rather than on the speed and reps.

At RKC courses, students often comment to the instructors, "You guys all stand the same way!" Like Russians. You will too. Whether you want to or not.

★ ★ ★

"IT'S YOUR FAULT": KETTLEBELL SAFETY 101

★ ★ ★

It's Your Fault.

—title of a future self-help book by
Rob Lawrence, Senior RKC

I t should be obvious to anyone but a complete moron that swinging a cast-iron ball the wrong way could lead to worse than a bad headache.

"Don't surf a tsunami!" No joke, the city of Malibu mailed a brochure with this warning to its residents. How stupid do you have to be, I wondered? Imagine my surprise when I read that more than 400 surfers had hit the waves in Hawaii, attracted by a tsunami warning, a few years back! Most of this stuff in this chapter is mind-numbingly obvious too, but in case you are one of those guys aspiring to win a Darwin Award, here it comes.

1. CHECK WITH DOCS
BEFORE YOU START TRAINING.

Especially an orthopedist and a cardiologist. The latter is no joking matter, since kettlebell training is unbelievably intense. Elsewhere in the book, you'll read how wrestler Michael Castrogiovanni got his heart rate to 211 BPM within minutes, although the "maximum heart rate" for his age group is only 195, and he was in stellar condition.

2. ALWAYS BE AWARE OF YOUR SURROUNDINGS.

Train in a place where there are no concerns about property damage or injury to anyone—including yourself.

"Train outside," insists Dan John. "You will NEVER reach your potential if you stay in the cozy confines of your gym... Grab a dumbbell or kettlebell . . . drive out to a nice spot, and simply invent a workout. Lift the thing as many ways as you can imagine and do as many reps as your body will allow."

Make sure to train on a flat surface; facing downhill invites back and knee problems.

As with basic range safety, make sure there are no comrades in the line of fire of your swings or snatches. The line is hot!

Is there anything to trip over? Including other kettlebells? —Clear out! At the RKC instructor courses, we drive the point home by punishing the students who get too close to parked kettlebells during wtheir sets.

How is the surface? If it is slippery or not flat—*move!* Dents left in the ground by kettlebells are something to watch out for as well. Following an RKC cert weekend, the football field we have trained on looks like Iraq after a U.S. air strike.

If you are training with ladies' light, rubberized kettlebells also make sure to choose a surface where they will not bounce.

Are you about to face the sun at the most challenging point of the get-up—if you are starting out facing a certain way?

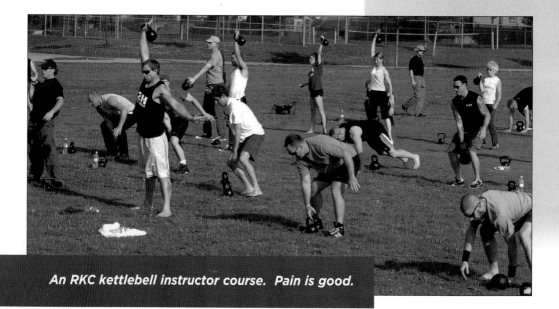

An RKC kettlebell instructor course. Pain is good.

3. WEAR AUTHORIZED SHOES.

Everything in this program must be practiced barefoot or in flat shoes without cushy soles. Wrestling shoes, work boots, tactical boots, and Converse Chuck Taylors are authorized. Almost any shoes worn by a guy named Chuck will do. Chuck #1, RKC, wears size 15 chicken-yellow water shoes, and Chuck #2, RKC, digs skateboard Vans with a chess print. Unconventional, but good enough not to warrant a set of push-ups.

Any sneakers a basketball player, runner, or aerobic instructor would wear are no good! Not only will the fancy shoes compromise your performance, they might set you up for a back or knee injury. I have explained the reasons why in *Power to the People!* so I will not repeat myself.

4. NEVER CONTEST FOR SPACE WITH A KETTLEBELL.

"Never contest for space with a kettlebell!" stresses Nate Morrison. "You will lose. Evade it and don't be where it wants to go."

If the bell wants to twist your elbow, shoulder, or any other joint in a way it is not supposed to go in our species, don't fight it. Abort! Guide the kettlebell to fall harmlessly, and move out of the way if necessary. Move those feet.

Better yet, anticipate the kettlebell's dynamics—to prevent problems instead of dealing with them.

5. PRACTICE ALL SAFETY MEASURES AT ALL TIMES.

Because "practice makes permanent," and "under stress we revert to training." How can you expect to do the right thing during the stressful last rep with a heavy kettlebell if you grooved wrong habits with the easy reps?

"As we continue to prove in the skydiving community," points out S.Sgt. Nate Morrison, USAF Pararescue, "it's the guys with the most jumps that seem to die for some very stupid reasons that are usually the result of being so familiar with a skill set that they go into automatic pilot mode ... Every time I jump ... I religiously check my [gear]. By the same token, every time I do a kettlebell windmill, I always follow a mental checklist, area is clear, snatch the bell, shift feet, look at the bell, inhale and pressurize for stability, the rear leg straight, the hip cocked back, descend under control, pause, return, lock out. Sounds like a lot, but it isn't, and I have never lost my balance under a KB of any size. My body appreciates this!"

The dumbest—and most common—injuries can be compared to safely navigating rush-hour traffic and then backing up into your mailbox.

A typical mistake is setting the kettlebell down sloppily, with a rounded back and the weight on the toes, following a hard (and often perfect) set of swings or snatches. Don't! Mentally stay with the set until the kettlebell is safely parked. Lower the kettlebell in a way you would if you were planning to do another rep. Then let go, and only then relax.

6. KEEP MOVING ONCE YOUR HEART RATE IS HIGH.

The need to warm up before exercise is an old wives' tale, but you do need a cool-down if you are coughing up a hairball. If you stand, sit, or lie down gasping for air following a hard set, your heart has to work unreasonably hard. You are still in severe oxygen debt, and moving your muscles—especially in the legs, by jogging, shadow boxing, even walking—pushes the blood back to the heart. Stop moving and your ticker has to work extra hard—too hard for some. Don't come to a complete stop until your heart rate and breathing are halfway down to normal.

Marty Gallagher makes a heart-rate monitor his only concession to hi-tech, in his "purposefully primitive" approach to strength and fitness. I have no experience with this tool, but when Marty speaks I listen. If you do get an HR monitor, you can also use it to watch out for overtraining. According to *Soldier, Be Strong!*, the Soviet armed forces manual, a 25–50 percent increase over the preworkout numbers is acceptable right after each session, but the heart rate is supposed to normalize within one to two hours.

7. BUILD UP THE TRAINING LOAD GRADUALLY USING COMMON SENSE, AND LISTEN TO YOUR BODY.

If you have sore elbows, it is your own fault, dude. Doing 50 cleans the first day you learned them was stupid.

"The training load" refers not only to the weight, sets, and reps, but also to the flexibility requirements. Don't force yourself into positions you are not ready for; develop your flexibility gradually. If you bang your forearm during cleans, don't go clean crazy until you have fixed your technique. Bruised and swollen forearms are signs of impatience, not toughness.

8. INSTRUCTION CANNOT COVER ALL CONTINGENCIES, AND THERE IS NO SUBSTITUTE FOR GOOD JUDGMENT.

And if you don't have good judgment, forget kettlebells and go take a Pilates class.

Now go back and read this chapter again. I feel your pain.

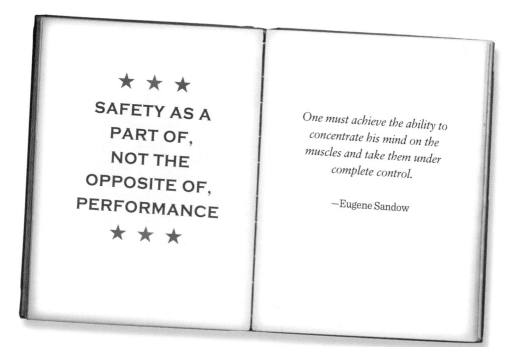

One must achieve the ability to concentrate his mind on the muscles and take them under complete control.

—Eugene Sandow

Physical culturist Eugene Sandow could do a back flip holding a 24-kilogram kettlebell in each hand, so he knew a thing or two about paying attention. It is not just about safety; it is about strength. At one of the RKC courses, senior instructor Rob Lawrence pointed out that in our system safety is viewed as a part of, not the opposite of, performance. Follow the instructions in this chapter, and not only will you drastically reduce your odds of getting hurt, with kettlebells or without, but you will get stronger—guaranteed.

1. HIPS FIRST!

A natural athlete moves from his hips, never from his back or knees. Hips-first movement is safest for your back and knees—and most powerful.

Stand up and place the edges of your hands into the creases on top of your thighs. Press your hands hard into

Physical culturist Eugene Sandow could do a back flip holding a 24-kilogram kettlebell in each hand, so he knew a thing or two about paying attention.

your "hinges" and stick your butt out while keeping your weight on your heels. I learned this neat trick from Kathy Foss Bakkum, RKC, God rest her strong and kind soul. It will teach you to go down by folding at your hip joints rather than bending through your back. Glenn Hyman, DC, RKC, stresses that this bit of instruction has been instrumental to the terrific success he has had rehabbing his patients with kettlebells.

Same thing on the way up: hips first. Drive with your glutes and hamstrings, less with your quads, and not at all with your back.

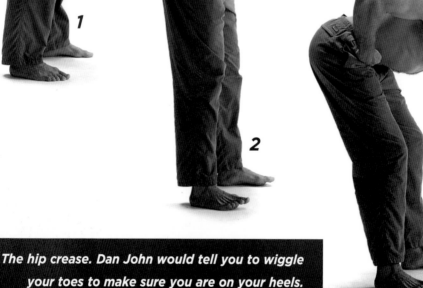

The hip crease. Dan John would tell you to wiggle your toes to make sure you are on your heels.

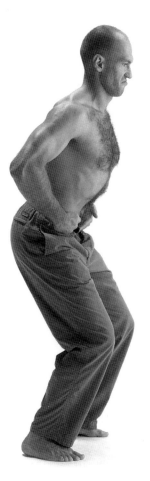

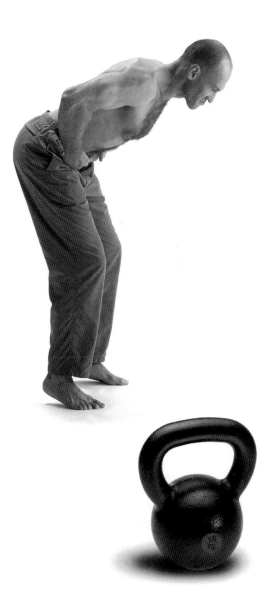

You have got to be kidding me, Comrade.
I said, fold at the hips. Not the spine, not the knees—
the hips!

2. DON'T SLOUCH. BEND BACK, NOT FORWARD, WHEN STRETCHING YOUR BACK.

A seemingly harmless thing to do is to slump forward after a kick-butt set or workout. Renowned physical therapist Robin McKenzie explains that most back pain is triggered by overstretching of the ligaments and the surrounding tissues. Which is in turn often caused by bad posture, especially the loss of the arch in the lower back. "After activity, the joints of the spine undergo a loosening process. If, after exercise, we place the back in an unsupported position for long periods, distortion within the joint readily occurs. This is true whether we sit in a slouched position or whether we stand, bending forward with our hands on our knees."

Avoid slouching, and perform five back bends immediately before and after lifting. "By standing upright and bending back before lifting," explains McKenzie, "you ensure that, as you begin the lift, there is no distortion already present in the joints of the lower back." Place your hands in the small of your back pointing your fingers downward and keep your legs straight. Bend back slowly using your hands as the fulcrum, pause for a second, and return to the upright position. Try to bend further with each successive rep.

Just because your back started hurting immediately following a given activity, you should not automatically blame the activity. Things are not always as they appear to be; most likely it was your slouch. So avoid slouching after vigorous exercise, and wrap up with the same five back bends.

Some Russian coaches have their athletes lie on their stomachs and read a book after a practice.

3. STAY TIGHT THROUGH YOUR WAIST.

"Stay tight"—maintain a tight muscle corset around your waist to protect your back. The abdomen should neither suck in nor protrude. Useful imagery is bracing for a punch (that can be arranged).

4. STAY LOOSE THROUGH YOUR ARMS.

Kettlebell cleans and snatches are not curls; the arms barely pass the force generated by the hips. Should your arms tense up, especially on the downswing, you are asking to tweak your elbows.

5. "TAME THE ARC."

We owe the "tame the arc" term to Senior RKC Rob Lawrence. This concept is best illustrated with Jeff Martone's hand-to-hand clean. Try it after you have learned the swing.

Pick up a kettlebell with one hand, and swing it between your legs. Flip the kettlebell and catch its round surface on your palm, the handle facing down. Keep your wrist tight. Press your upper arm against your body, keep your elbow low. Don't lean back.

Drop the kettlebell between your legs—watch your knees—catch the handle, and repeat.

Very quickly, you will realize that swinging the kettlebell in a big arc gives you problems. The bell escapes forward away from you and either pulls you forward or simply does not allow you to palm it. Swinging the bell too high is just as annoying.

Tame the arc and your problems are solved. On the way down, it is done by tossing the kettlebell back rather than down, so your forearm almost hits you in the groin. "Hike pass." On the way up, the answer is *not* pulling with the biceps but rather yanking the shoulder back, like starting a lawn mower.

Taming the arc also applies to racking the kettlebell on your chest after a clean or catching it overhead after a snatch. Letting the kettlebell travel in a big arc means banging yourself on the forearm. Tightening the arc by outrunning the kettlebell with your fist makes the catch soft.

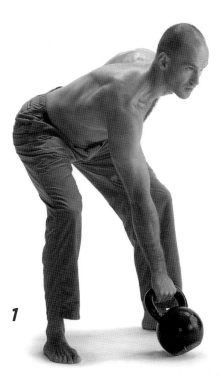

1

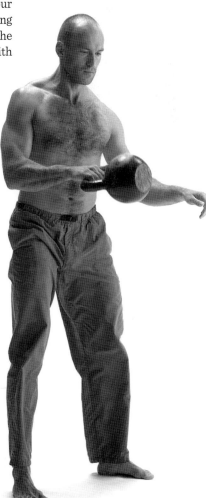

2

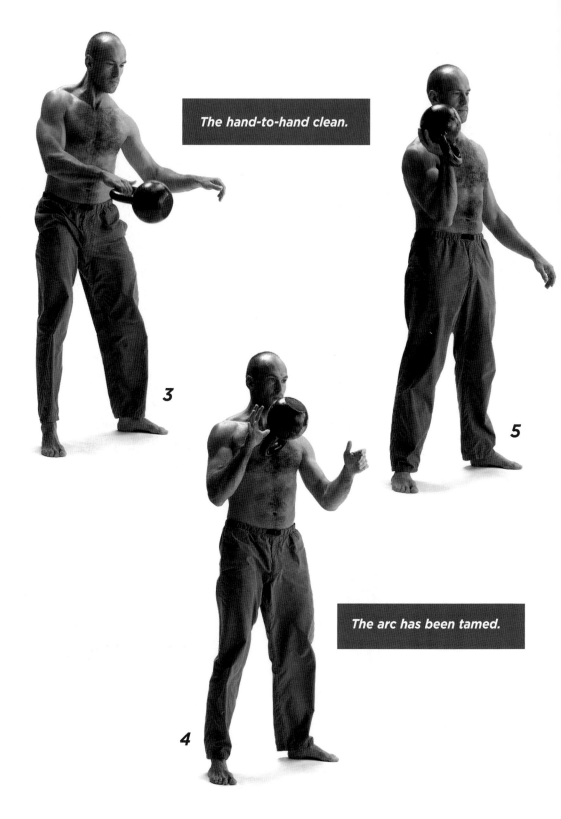

The hand-to-hand clean.

3

5

4

The arc has been tamed.

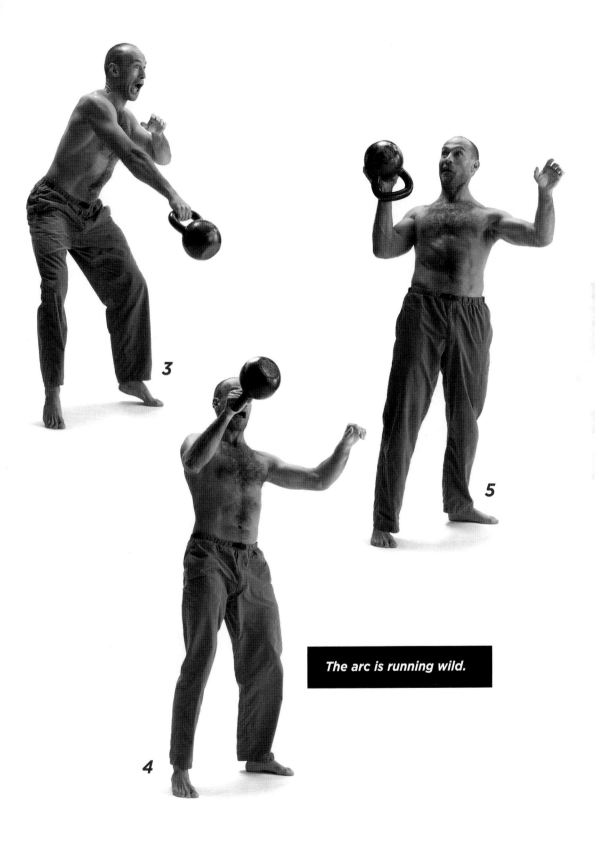

3

4

5

The arc is running wild.

6. KEEP YOUR SHOULDERS IN THEIR SOCKETS.

Old-time world wrestling champion and girevik extraordinaire Ivan Shemyakin could do one-legged jumps holding a seven-*pood* barbell overhead! Apart from great leg power, this feat required the strength and skill to lock out the elbows and retract the shoulders at the instant of every impact. Put up a very light kettlebell or dumbbell overhead and walk fast or even jump. You will quickly learn that your shoulder and elbow do not care for this—unless you lock your elbow and suck your shoulder into its socket every time you get jarred.

The lesson: pull your shoulder into your body the way a turtle pulls in its head when you are supporting the kettlebell overhead.

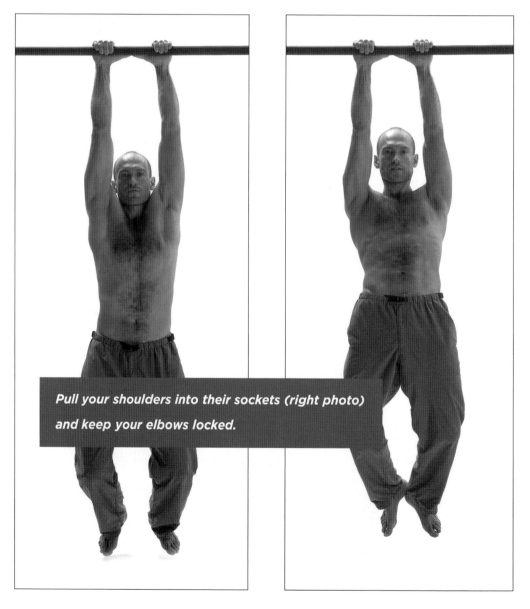

Pull your shoulders into their sockets (right photo) and keep your elbows locked.

Senior RKC Steve Cotter teaches the following shoulder retraction drill: Lie on your back and raise your straight arm. Have your training partner carefully pull up on the arm until it starts "separating" from your body. The second time, suck the arm into the shoulder socket and have him pull again. If you have retracted correctly, the arm will stay "connected" to the body, and your friend will lift your body off the deck.

If you train alone, do the pull-up bar drill by Anthony Diluglio, RKC. Hang on a pull-up bar. Use a narrow, overhand grip. Flex your triceps and pull yourself up an inch or two by retracting your arms into your body like a turtle's head. Don't bend your arms; just pull your shoulders into their sockets. And pull your shoulder blades together.

By the way, note how your arms stay close to your ears. This is the way they should be when you hold kettlebells overhead.

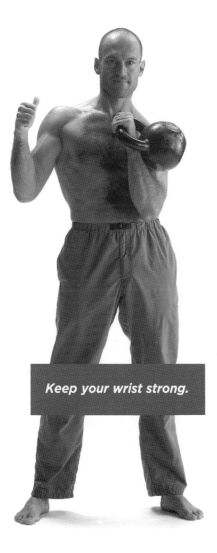

Keep your wrist strong.

7. DON'T HYPEREXTEND YOUR WRISTS.

The heavy kettlebell is determined to bend your wrist backward. Don't let it happen! Stick your hand far inside the handle so the weight rests on the heel of your palm. Then counter with the wrist flexors, the muscles that gooseneck your wrist.

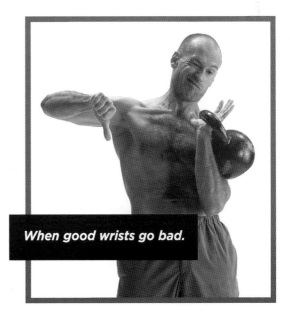

When good wrists go bad.

8. Keep your elbows straight.

This rule applies to two points in the kettlebell's flight plan, on the bottom of the downswing and at the overhead lockout. The purpose is giving your elbows a break.

For mysterious reasons, locking out the joints—extending, not hyperextending—is a taboo is Western gyms. A personal trainer who cannot even straighten out his arms without any weight warns his clients that they will "hurt their joints" if they lock them out. A muscle-bound idiot.

Without going into boring details (ask your chiropractor), the inability to straighten out the elbow when holding a weight overhead often leads to problems upstream—in the shoulder. So straighten it out, Comrade, dude, dudette!

And failing to let the elbow go completely straight once you have dropped the kettlebell between your legs is murder on the elbow.

9. Take care of your hands.

Ripped calluses are manly, but since they make you lose training time, try to avoid them when you do your quick lifts.

It is elementary, Watson—you must gradually build up the volume of swings, cleans, and snatches to let your skin adapt.

You may want to sandpaper your kettlebell's handles, as kettlebell sport competitors do. Remove the paint and smooth out the iron.

Unlike presses and other grind lifts, swings, cleans, and snatches call for a loose grip. "Hook" the handle with your fingers rather than gripping it.

Try to lift in a way that minimally stretches the skin on your palm. Figure it out.

Load the calluses at the bases of your fingers as little as possible; let the kettlebell handle glide from the "hook" of the fingers to the heel of the palm and back in a manner that does not pinch the skin at the bases of the fingers.

Do not let the calluses get thick and rough. Russian gireviks soak their hands in hot water at night, then thin out and smooth out their calluses with a pumice stone, and finally apply an oily cream or a three-to-one mix of glycerin and ammonia. I hang my head in shame to be giving you metrosexual skin-care advice.

Speaks Brett Jones, Senior RKC, who gives his hands the double abuse of kettlebell lifting and extreme gripping feats:

"Go out and get Cornhuskers Lotion and use it several times a day. This lotion is unique in that it is not greasy and actually toughens and conditions your skin. At night you may want to use a product that penetrates and moisturizes in a different way. Bag Balm and other heavy (oily) lotions can be used at night and can best be absorbed if you put them on before bed and wear mittens, socks or specially designed gloves available at some health and beauty stores. [Brett, I will take your word for it.]

"File or shave off your calluses. By using an Emery board, buffing pad, or even high grade sand paper you can simply file off the excess callous so that it never gets thick enough to tear or rip. There are even callous shavers available that use a razor blade with a guide to shave off thick calluses. But, if you file often and correctly you may never need them. You do not want to file away the entire callous. The thickened part that becomes 'caught' or pinched during the snatches or KB work is what you should file off. Your calluses are there for a reason. Just keep them in check to reduce the possibility for tears.

"Listen to your hands. If your skin begins to pull, tingle or give indications of a blister or tear, listen to it and stop. Halting a set early to save your hands is far preferable to ignoring the warning and allowing a tear to occur which can derail your training."

Mark Reifkind, RKC, a man who has been hard on his hands with gymnastics, powerlifting, and now kettlebells, recommends "a technique I used back in gymnastics to deal with overly thick and hard calluses.

1) Soak the hands in hot water for at least five minutes. Hot baths work well but showers take forever.

2) Dry the hands and wait 30 seconds or so for the blood to come back.

3) Sand the hand with pumice stone or sandpaper callous remover.

The skin just sloughs off with very little effort and all the pads get nice and flat. Just enough to protect but not tear."

Rif will also tell you what to do if you have gone too far and got blisters:

"What I do is cut the dead skin away and as close to the remaining callous pad as possible. Clean and dry and then place a square of athletic tape (MUST be porous or it won't work) over the tear and work it into the skin until it is seamless. Leave it on until it gets wet or dirty then replace. If the tape won't stick it is wet or dirty.

"This technique allows the tear to get air so it will dry out but the porous covering allows it to be just moist enough so you don't get cracks in the center. Works every time. You can work out with the square of tape covering the tear."

If your workout calls for snatches but your paws feel like they are ready to pop, do two-handed swings instead to minimize the stress on the skin of the hands.

A special note on training in high humidity. Rob Lawrence, Senior RKC, advises, "When you are working out under humid conditions, the deadweight snatch is your friend. You can do multiple sets without ripping your hands. Snatch the weight, lower to shoulder, lower to ground, repeat."

The backswing, and thus most of the skin stress, is eliminated. You could do the dead snatch even if the weather is dry but your hands are raw.

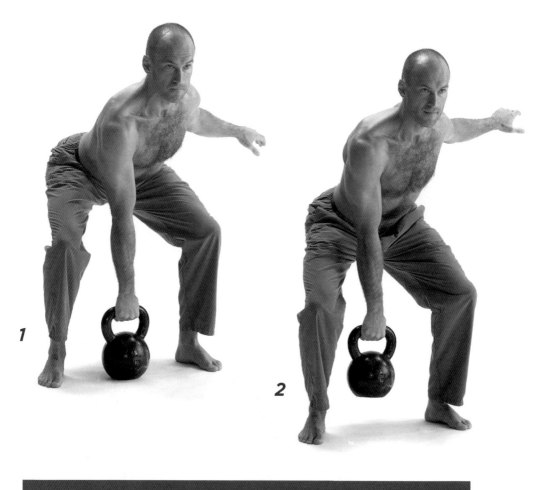

The dead snatch resembles the snatch from Olympic weightlifting.

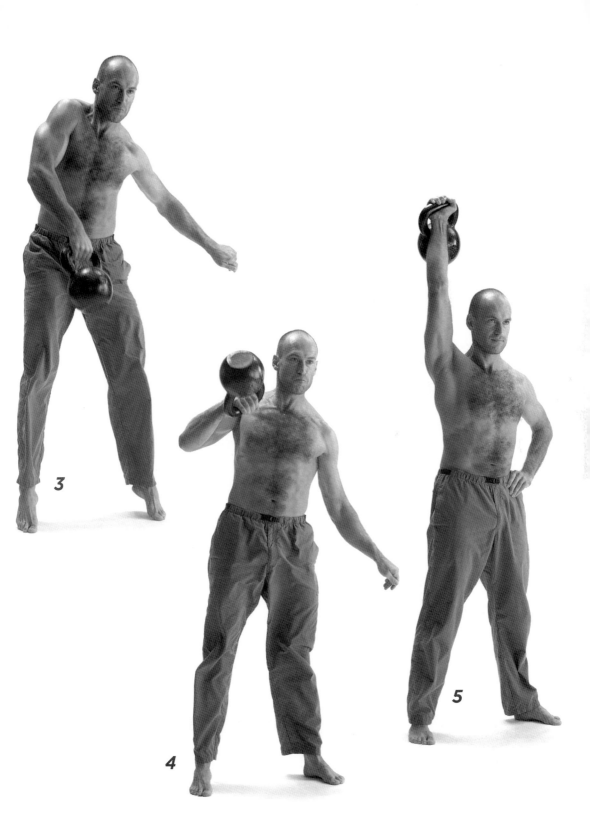

3

4

5

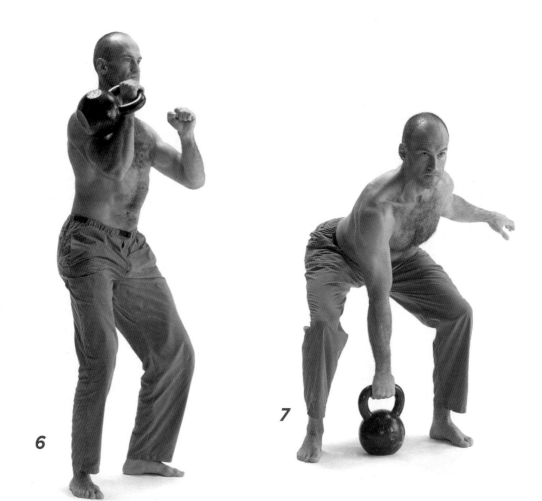

6

7

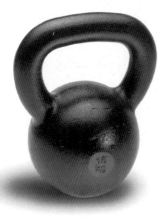

Before you touch a kettlebell, make sure to reread this chapter many times. Ideally before bedtime. Like the Russian military regulations, full of exciting trivia such as the dimensions of the guard tower or the maximum allowed height of the grass around it, it will assure deep, sound sleep within 15 minutes.

THE NEW RKC
PROGRAM MINIMUM

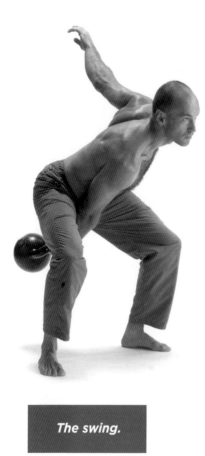

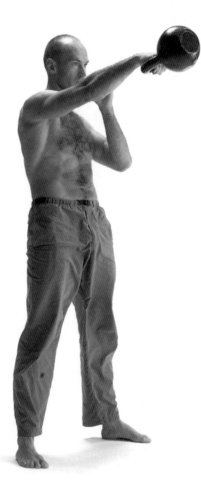

The swing.

CHAPTER 2:

The New RKC Program Minimum

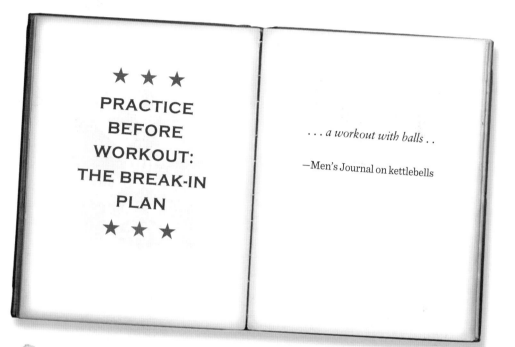

★ ★ ★

PRACTICE
BEFORE
WORKOUT:
THE BREAK-IN
PLAN

★ ★ ★

. . . a workout with balls . .

—Men's Journal on kettlebells

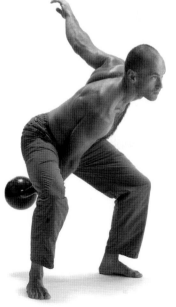

T ime to hit the metal. You will start your desissification with patient practice of two staples of the Russian Kettlebell Challenge, the swing and the get-up.

The swing is what its name implies—you are swinging a kettlebell from between your legs up to your chest level and back, using your hips to power the movement, as you would if you were jumping.

The get-up, introduced into the system by Steve Maxwell, Senior RKC, is just as aptly named. Start out lying on your back holding a kettlebell up with a straight arm, as if you have just finished a one-arm bench press.

Without jerking or unlocking the elbow, stand up and then slowly lie back down. Although the elbow does not bend whatsoever for the duration of the set, the get-up can be wiggled into the "press" category, because the static overload of holding a weight overhead, surprisingly, builds pressing strength.

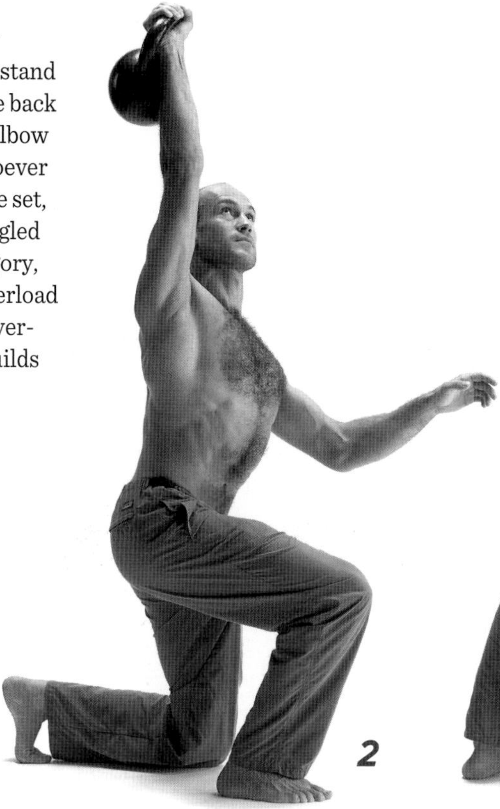

2

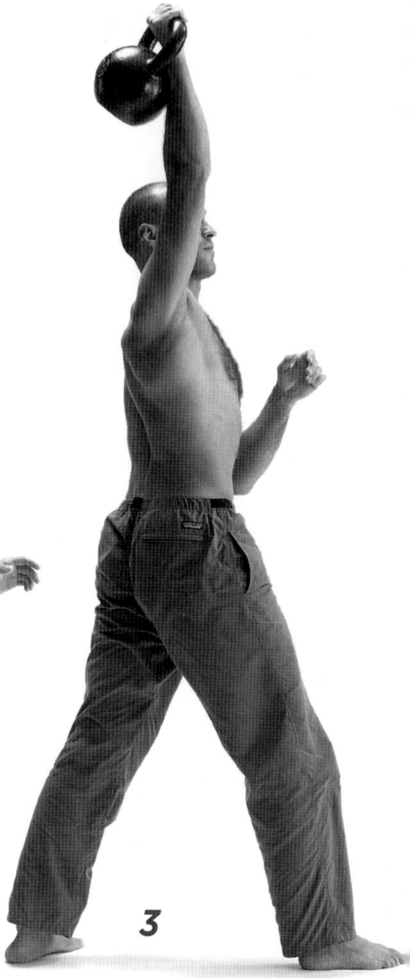

3

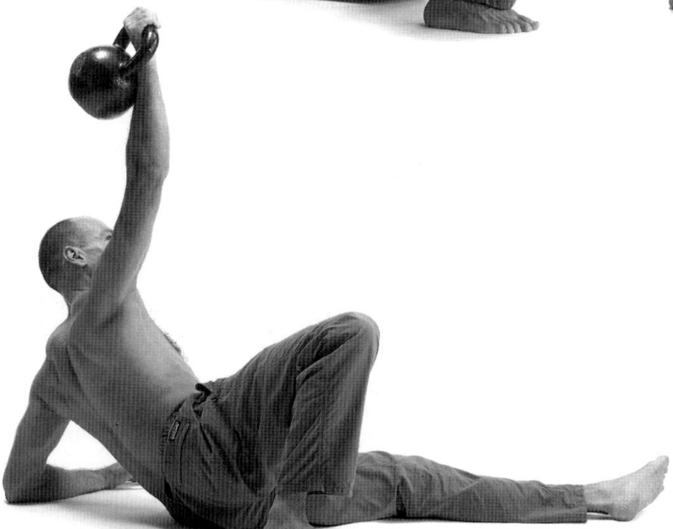

1

Study the safety chapters and the descriptions of the swing and the get-up. Watch the Enter the Kettlebell! DVD many times. Then practice these two exercises and their remedial drills almost daily, and at least three times a week. Practice; don't work out! The same way you would practice shooting a pistol, stop before your fragile skill goes to pot and the target becomes a blur. Do a couple of reps of one drill, rest, do a few reps of the other, rest some more, do a remedial drill, and so on. Keep reading the exercise descriptions or watching the DVD over and over when you are resting. Look for subtleties, use your highlighter, take notes.

Don't try to get yourself smoked; this will come soon enough. A 30-minute practice is about right. When done, you should feel energized rather than wiped out. You should hardly be sore the day after.

Stay on the above break-in program for as long as it takes. Have patience—you are taking on a challenging skill set, akin to a martial art.

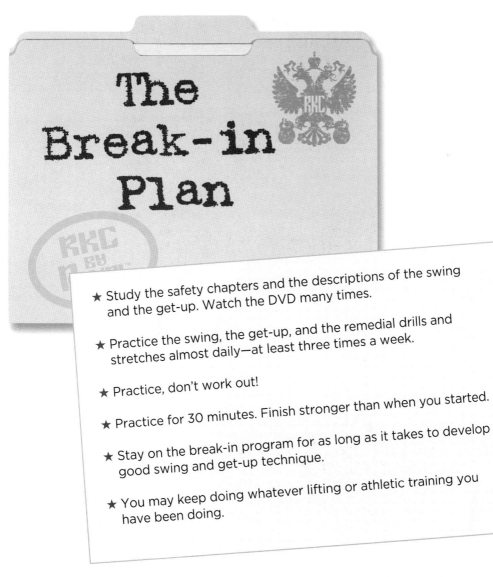

The Break-in Plan

★ Study the safety chapters and the descriptions of the swing and the get-up. Watch the DVD many times.

★ Practice the swing, the get-up, and the remedial drills and stretches almost daily—at least three times a week.

★ Practice, don't work out!

★ Practice for 30 minutes. Finish stronger than when you started.

★ Stay on the break-in program for as long as it takes to develop good swing and get-up technique.

★ You may keep doing whatever lifting or athletic training you have been doing.

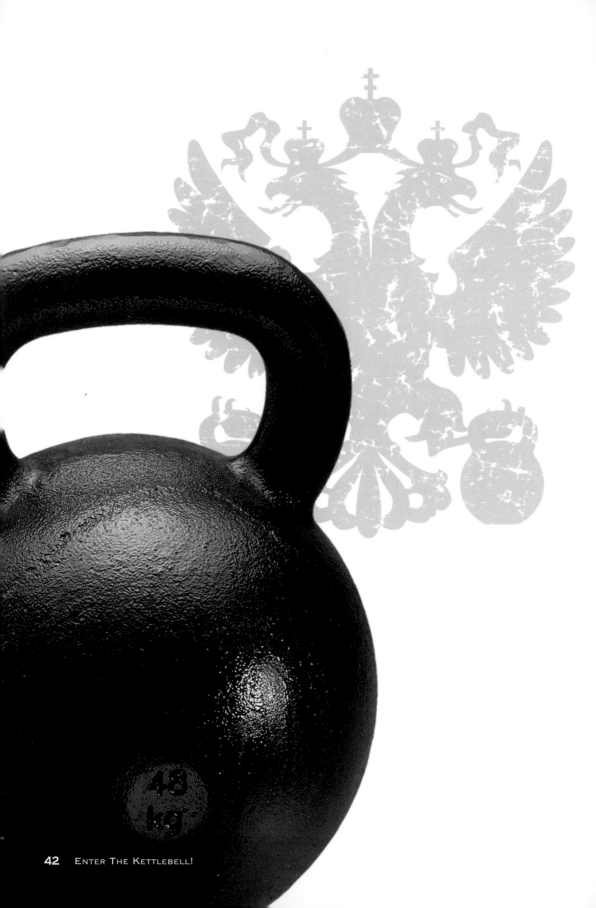

★ ★ ★

THE SWING—
FOR LEGS AND
CONDITIONING
THAT WON'T
GIVE UP

★ ★ ★

*Kettlebell high-rep ballistics
are the closest
you can get to fighting
without throwing a punch*

—A federal counterterrorist
operator

I dare you to find a single exercise, kettlebell or not, that delivers more benefits than the kettlebell swing! Senior RKC instructor Steve Maxwell, a Brazilian Jiu-jitsu World Champion, has flat-out stated that doing the perfect kettlebell swing alone is superior to 99 percent of the sophisticated strength and conditioning programs out there.

The swing is exactly what its name implies: a swing of a kettlebell from between your legs up to your chest level. The arms stay straight but loose; the power is generated by the hips. The motion is akin to the standing vertical jump, except the energy is projected into the kettlebell rather than being used to lift the body.

1

TASK: SWING

Condition:
Swing a kettlebell between your legs and then in front of you up to the chest level for repetitions.

The swing.

2

3

Standard:

1. Maintain the box-squat alignment during swings and when picking up or setting down
   the kettlebell:
   - a) keep your head up;
   - b) keep a straight—not to be confused with "upright"—back;
   - c) sit back rather than dip down.
2. Extend the hips and knees fully on the top: the body must form a straight line.
3. The kettlebell must form an extension of the straight and loose arm(s) on the
   top of the swing.

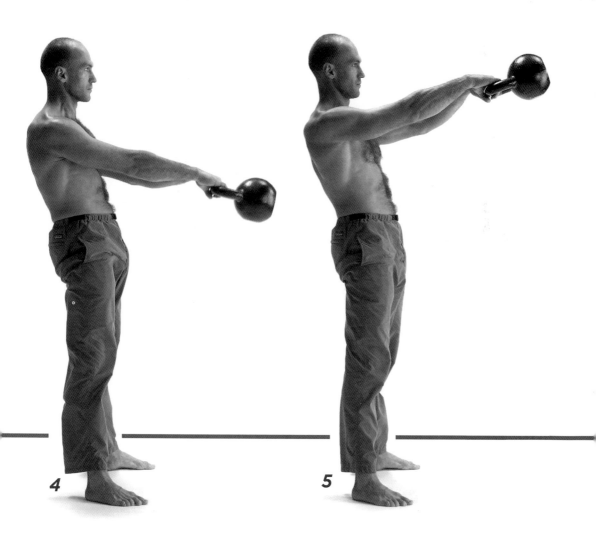

4

5

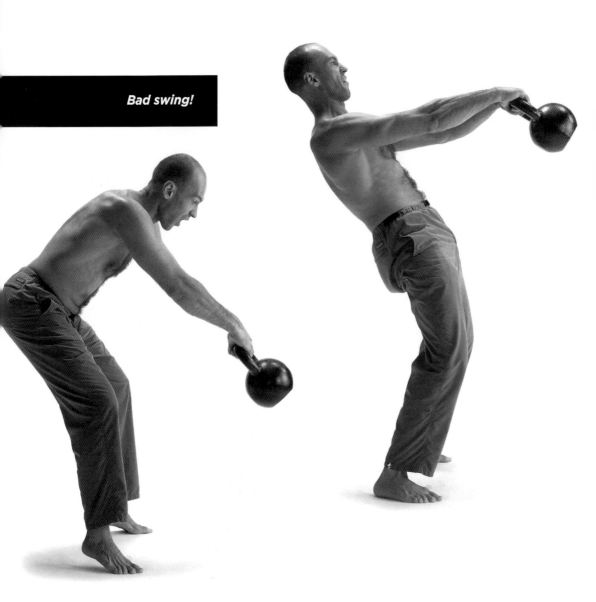

SWING MASTERY STEP #1: THE BOX SQUAT

The box squat is just like sitting down on a chair or a curb. Powerlifters invented this drill to improve their squatting depth, flexibility, technique, and power. It will serve you well.

First let us revisit the hip-crease drill. Stand up and place the edges of your hands into the creases on top of your thighs. Press your hands hard into your hinges and stick your butt out while keeping your weight on your heels. You should feel the muscles in your hinges, the hip flexors, tighten up as if you are doing sit-ups.

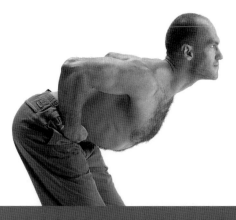

Press your hands hard into your hinges and stick your butt out while keeping your weight on your heels.

Now pick up a kettlebell and hold it in front of you by its horns. You need it for balance, at least in the beginning. Stand a foot or so in front of a sturdy bench or box facing away from it. Crease at your hips and push your butt back.

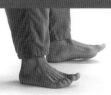

You may hold a kettlebell for balance.

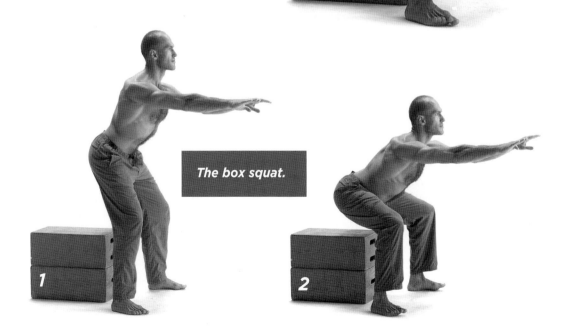

The box squat.

1

2

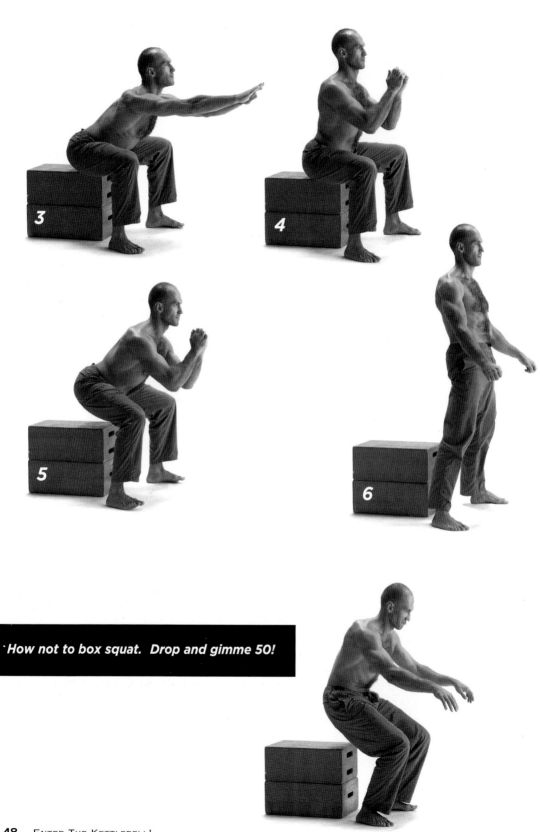

How not to box squat. Drop and gimme 50!

Keep pushing your rear end back. Your knees will bend, but only as an afterthought. Hips first!

Don't let your knees go forward. Ideally, your shins should be close to vertical. If you do not feel your hamstrings tighten up when you descend, you are squatting wrong. Imagine that you are wearing ski boots and your ankles cannot bend. If you own a pair, why imagine? Wear them. You cannot help but learn to fold in your hip joints.

Never let your knees bow in. The knees should track the feet, and the feet should be pointing slightly outward.

The movement is similar to the face-the-wall squat, except your butt is sticking out and your body is folded forward more.

Push the kettlebell forward to counterbalance, and keep sitting back.

Back, not down.

Keep sitting back until your backside softly touches down on the box. You must not fall even an inch! Control your descent all the way! You will feel tightness on the top of your thighs and a stretch in your hamstrings if you do it right.

Time to get up.

Rock back. Instantly rock forward and stand up while observing the following rules:

First, do not cross your ankles or push your feet underneath you. Plant your feet like you mean it, with your shins almost upright. Remember that you are stuck in cement up to your knees.

Second, fold over and reach forward. If you have set your feet far enough forward as instructed, trying to stand up while remaining upright is an exercise in futility, a challenge to the fundamental laws of physics.

The moment you feel that your weight has loaded your feet, push your feet hard straight down into the ground.

Tense your glutes—pinch a coin—and drive your hips forward until you stand up. Lock out your knees by pulling up your kneecaps. Lock out your hips by cramping the glutes. Do not even think about scooping forward! Your knees will slip forward only if you completely disregard the instructions. Drop and give me 50! Then get someone to restrain your shins by hand.

If the technique instruction for the box squat seems exhaustive, please realize that attention to details is what makes this, or any other effective program, work. Anything worth doing is worth doing right. Besides, once you get the box squat down pat, most of the remaining drills will build on its foundation and will be a piece of cake to learn and master.

SWING MASTERY STEP #2:
THE BOX SQUAT TO A VERTICAL JUMP

Box squat by the book then rock forward and jump straight up! The expert vertical jump is just like the kettlebell swing, clean, or snatch: the hips are aggressively stretch-loaded at the start and drive hard all the way to the top. Do a few. Feel the power. Don't start swings until your jumps are crisp and aggressive.

Once you have your jumps dialed in, the swing will be a piece of *pirogi*.

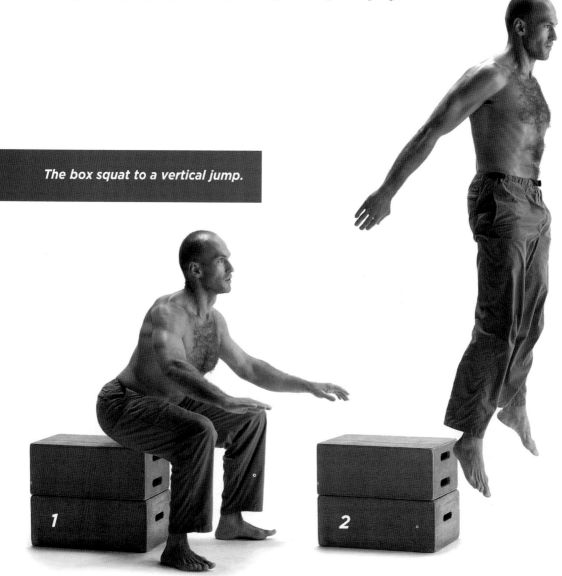

The box squat to a vertical jump.

SWING MASTERY STEP #3: THE TOWEL SWING

At the RKC think tank, we are relentless about streamlining our teaching. As of today, the towel swing drill from Stephen Troy, RKC, a full-contact karate fighter from Chicago, takes the cake for getting the most technique out of the victim with the least instruction.

"When you're using your hips to drive up the kettlebell on the swing, your arms should just be ropes attached to the bell," explains Troy. "That means the bell should project out straight from your arms throughout its arc. Many beginning lifters, and especially guys with big chests, have a hard time not flexing them when swinging a kettlebell, and as a result they sometimes rely too much on upper body strength to bring up the bell.

"To make sure you're swinging without using your arms, attach a lifting strap or very short rope [or a towel] to a kettlebell...

"Try a few swings. If you're driving the weight up with your hips, the bell, rope, and arm should all be in one line throughout the rep. If you're using your arms, your hands will rise up above the strap and bell."

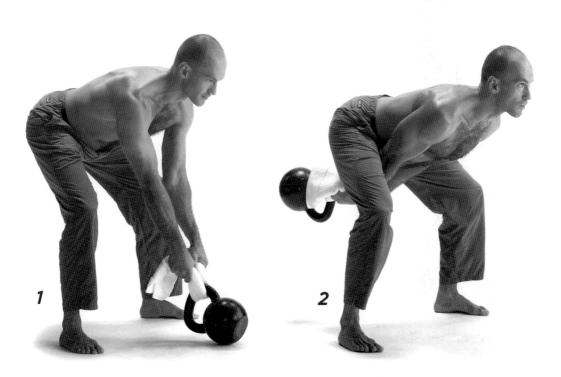

The towel swing is the same as the regular swing, except for the fact that the kettlebell hangs on a towel that you are holding with both hands. The towel will exaggerate your mistakes, provide you with feedback, and teach you how to swing right—in minutes.

In a nutshell, swing the kettlebell back between your legs—think "hike pass" from football—and then in front of you. The classic swing is done to the chest level, but there is no need to be so picky at this point. Keep your arms and shoulders relaxed; drive with the hips. Even during the hike pass, emphasize the hips, not the arms. "Throw" the kettlebell by hinging aggressively, as if you are descending into an explosive box squat.

Snap the hips and straighten out—but don't hyperextend—the knees.

The towel swing.

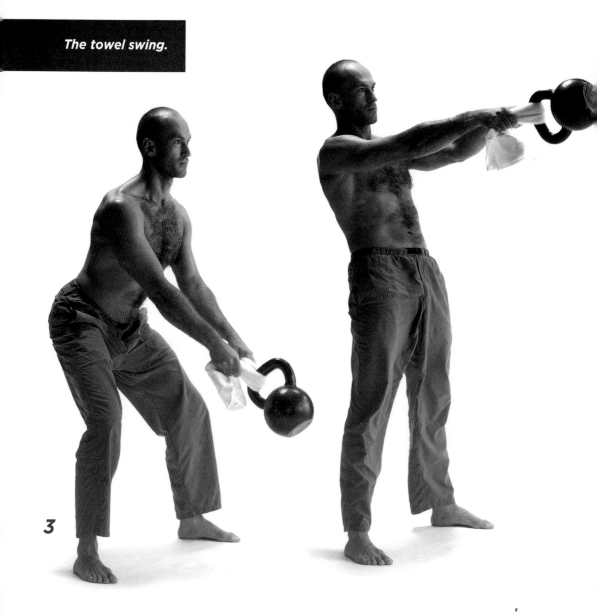

3

Again, the knees go up, not back. Pull up your kneecaps.

All of the sumo deadlift checkpoints apply (see Chapter 1).

Start swinging! If you have messed up a rep and the kettlebell is pulling you forward so that you are about to lose balance, drop it!

Don't hold your breath. I am not going to tell you how to breathe at this point of the game, just breathe. Ideally, in sync with the movement.

The beauty of the towel swing is the clear feedback it provides. Even if you do not know exactly what you should change, you will figure it out through trial and error by trying to make your arms, the towel, and the kettlebell line up. Don't forget to line up your whole body as well as you did in the dead lift and the vertical jump.

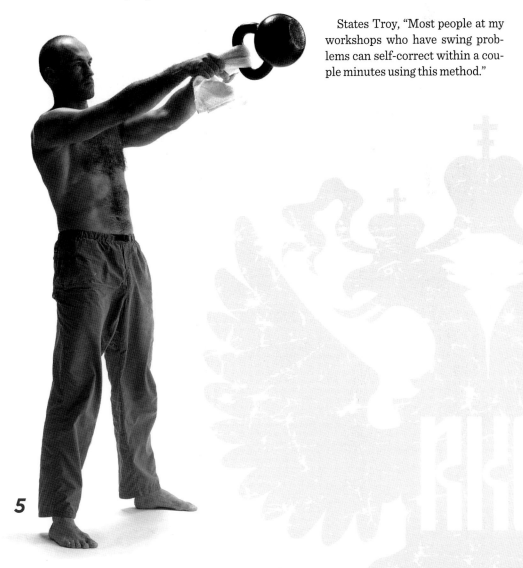

States Troy, "Most people at my workshops who have swing problems can self-correct within a couple minutes using this method."

5

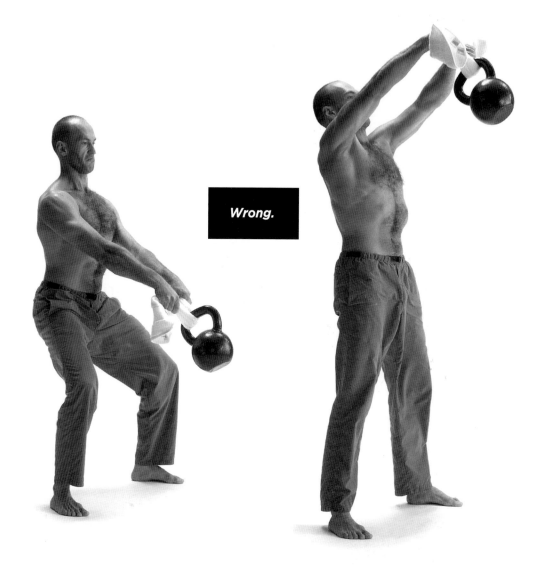

Wrong.

DO YOU HAVE TWO STRAIGHT LINES ON THE TOP OF YOUR SWING?

★ Your arms—the towel —the kettlebell

★ Your legs—your upper body—your head

Once you have succeeded in making these two straight lines, you are ready for the regular swing.

But better finesse your timing first. You will soon notice that there is a time lag between the driving force of the hips and the kettlebell's flight—like in a punch. The towel reveals this important subtlety of the swing. Keep swinging, and pay attention to the timing of your efforts. Try to make the kettlebell hover weightless for a moment at the apex.

Drive your hips explosively, but don't rush the kettlebell. Let it catch up as your hip drive goes up your body like a wave. Hurrying the kettlebell is like punching with the arm—ineffective.

Work some more on your timing. Try to make the kettlebell go a certain height between your waist and your head without scooping your body or pulling with your arms.

Swing Mastery Step #4: The Swing Proper

Once you have the towel swing licked, you are ready for the regular swing. Stand a foot or so behind your kettlebell, sit back, and take a hold of the handle with both hands. While keeping your weight on your heels—important!—hike pass the kettlebell behind you, fairly close to your groin. Drive the hips through and start swinging.

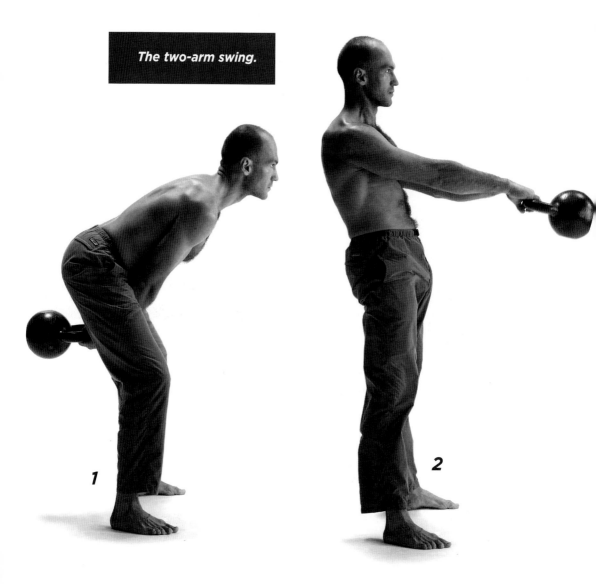

The two-arm swing.

1

2

This is a good time to get your breathing right. On the top of each swing, loudly call out the number of each rep. True, it is not easy to say "one hundred twenty-seven" quickly enough, but by the time your reps get that high you will have synced your breathing, so you may shut up. I insist.

What you are shooting for, eventually, are sharp exhalations synchronized with the finish of each swing. This is the way martial artists and boxers breathe when they punch. Note that you should never blow out all of your air, as this makes you weak and your back vulnerable. The amount of your breath that comes out with a grunt is just right.

Sharply inhale through your nose when the kettlebell has almost bottomed out behind your legs. It will not be easy in the beginning, but it will come if you call out your rep numbers on the top.

When you are done with your set, pay attention to how you park the kettlebell. Following the backswing, let the bell passively swing forward slightly and set it down between your feet. Don't round your back or roll forward on your toes! Don't relax until the bell is safely parked.

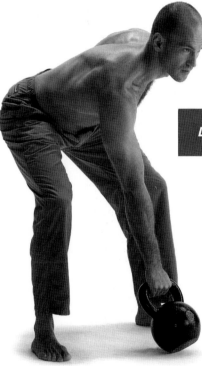

Don't relax until the bell is safely parked.

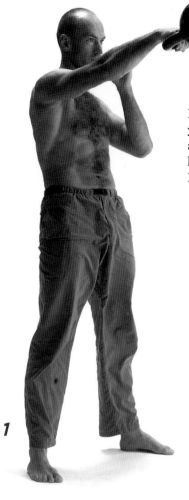

When you feel ready, move up to the one-arm swing. Don't grip the kettlebell's handle, but rather hook it with your fingers. Try to keep your arm and shoulder as relaxed as possible—remember the rope analogy. Keep your other hand clear; don't get cute by pushing off your knee! Big Brother is watching.

1

The one-arm swing.

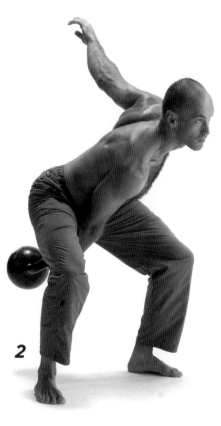

2

Soon you will progress to the hand-to-hand swing. Release the kettlebell on the top of the swing, and pluck it out of the air with your other hand. If you have swung the kettlebell too far and you have to reach forward to grab it, just let it go! Your back will thank you.

Move crisply, like a karate punch.

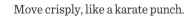

1

2

3

The hand-to-hand swing.

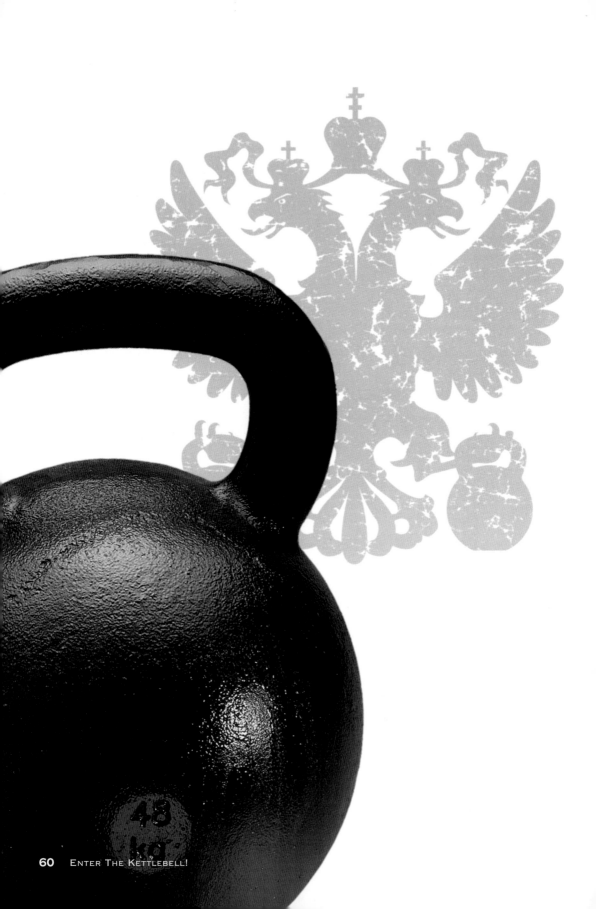

★ ★ ★

THE GET-UP
–FOR SHOULDERS
THAT CAN
TAKE
PUNISHMENT
AND DISH IT OUT

★ ★ ★

The one-arm get-up is a general test of strength which had considerable appeal to most strongmen of yesteryear. . . . It has always made a hit with the theatrical public, for it was obvious to them that magnificent strength was being displayed when an athlete did a one-arm get-up with a heavy bell.

—Siegmund Klein,
an American strength legend

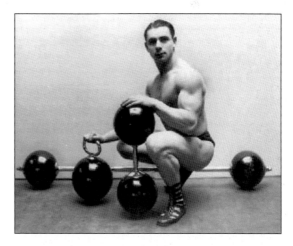

The kettlebell get-up is responsible for many miraculous shoulder comebacks in our community. Many hard men with high mileage—who were ready to hang up their spurs and take up golf—got to stay in the fight.

In addition to developing spectacular shoulder mobility and stability, both essential for taking the punishment of fighting and sports, the get-up molds the strength to dish punishment out. Our resident kettlebell press expert, Senior RKC Mike Mahler, saw his big press get even bigger once he started doing heavy get-ups. And when Brett Jones, Senior RKC, started doing get-ups with "the Beast," the 106-pound kettlebell, his impressive military pressing strength immediately shot up as well.

TASK: GET-UP

Condition:
Lie on your back, pick up the kettlebell with both hands, and press it with one. Slowly stand up while keeping your working arm straight and vertical. Assist yourself by pushing into the ground with the free arm. Slowly reverse the movement.

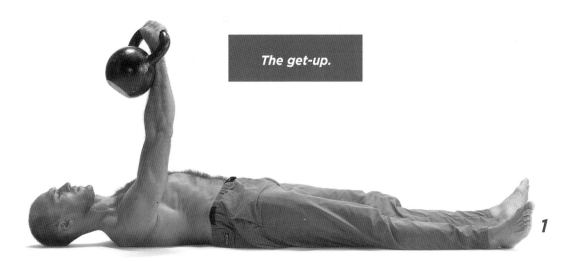

The get-up.

1

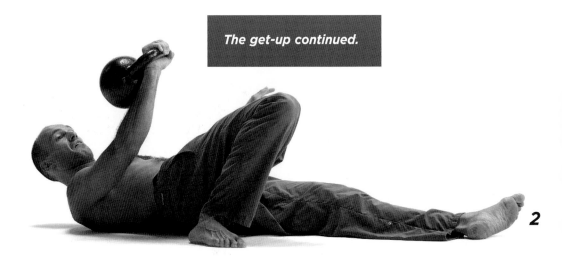

The get-up continued.

2

Standard:

1. Use both hands to lift the kettlebell from the ground at the start of the exercise and to return it to the ground at the finish (an elbow safety measure).
2. At no point allow the kettlebell to hyperextend and stress the wrist. Keep the handle at the base of the palm and keep your wrist tight.
3. Lock your elbow and keep it locked for the duration of the set.
4. Keep your shoulder in its socket, especially during movement transitions.
5. Get up and down seamlessly, without jerky transitions.
6. Don't do anything that you would not or could not do with a very heavy kettlebell. That implies keeping your arm vertical and totally controlling the kettlebell and your whole body at all times.

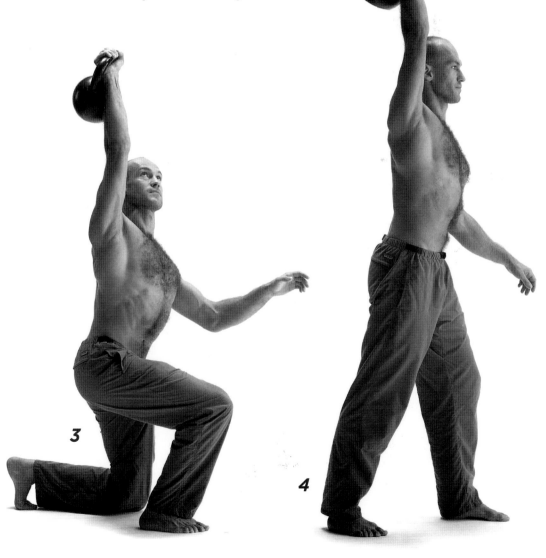

3

4

GET-UP MASTERY STEP #1: PICK YOUR KETTLEBELL UP AND SET IT DOWN SAFELY

Before standing up with a kettlebell, you need to pick it up from the ground. Recall one of the Kettlebell Safety 101 rules: "Don't do anything you couldn't or wouldn't do with a very heavy kettlebell." Then conduct a mental experiment: what would happen if you were to lie down on your back and try to pick up a 106-pounder lying at your side with one hand? Unless you are familiar with the arm-wrestling "post-up" technique, you will strain the inside of your elbow. Which is why we pick the kettlebell up with both hands.

You are about to do a right handed get-up. With the kettlebell sitting on your right next to your ribs, curl grip the handle with your right hand, then overlap your fingers with a thumbless grip of your left. Keeping the kettlebell as close to your body as possible, bring it to your chest with this two-handed pistol grip. Let go with the left.

Roll onto your right side and spear your right hand deep inside the handle. Gooseneck your wrist slightly to counter the kettlebell's determination to hyperextend your wrist. Grip the handle moderately. Keep it that way for the duration.

Press the kettlebell above your chest with your right. Keep your shoulder down, toward the ground and toward your feet.

Make sure to repeat the sequence in reverse on the way down. Overgrip the working hand with your free hand, lower the kettlebell to your chest, then roll onto your side and release the kettlebell once it is on the ground. Not sooner!

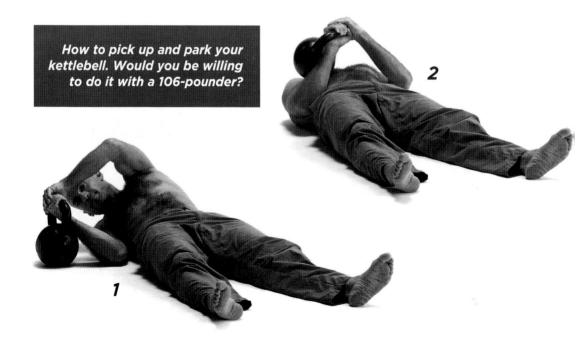

How to pick up and park your kettlebell. Would you be willing to do it with a 106-pounder?

2

1

GET-UP MASTERY STEP #2: KEEP YOUR ELBOW STRAIGHT AND YOUR SHOULDER IN ITS SOCKET

A great visualization comes from Iyengar Yoga. Visualize "a power source" in the locked elbow. It sends energy up the forearm and down into the shoulder. Simultaneously, the arm is "growing longer" toward the kettlebell and "pressing hard into the shoulder socket." Keep that image throughout the get-up and the "get-down."

GET-UP MASTERY STEP #3: THE HALF GET-UP

Bend your right knee and plant your foot. Pushing off your right foot and propping yourself with your left elbow (Josh Henkin, RKC, says you should "pivot" on your elbow), slowly sit up. Keep your arm straight and vertical and your eyes on the kettlebell. Keep your shoulder in its socket! Breathe shallowly while keeping your stomach tight throughout the rep.

A sit-up is good enough for the first rep. Slowly reverse the sequence. Don't hit the ground hard—you could end up with a kettlebell stuck in your grill!

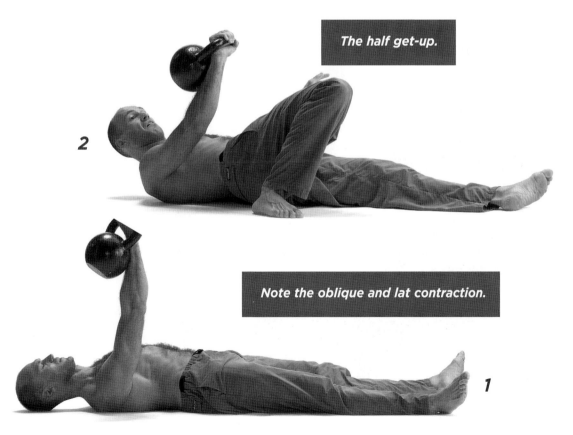

The half get-up.

2

Note the oblique and lat contraction.

1

A few years ago we taught an RKC instructor course to a detail of bodyguards working under an ex-Delta Force operator for one of Mexico's largest companies. One of our students, Mario, doubled as one of Mexico's highest-ranked kickboxers and a physical therapist. We heard from him some time later. Mario had fixed many ruined shoulders using just the start of the get-up—a half sit-up with a pivot on the opposite elbow.

3

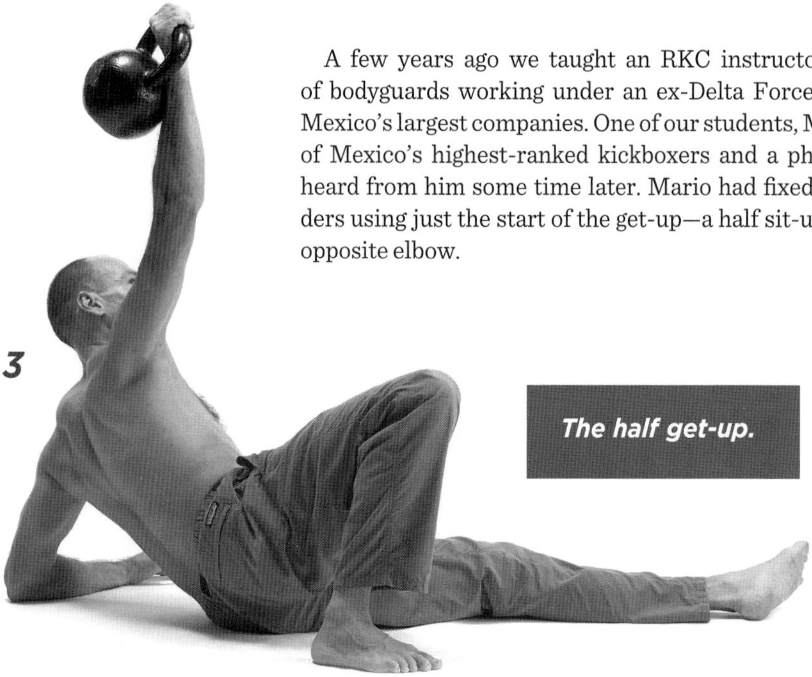

The half get-up.

GET-UP MASTERY STEP #4: THE GET-UP ALL THE WAY

Once you have succeeded in sitting up, stand up. Do it any safe way you want to; the important thing is to keep the movement smooth and seamless. No jerking as you are making transitions.

Doing a full get-up by the book, the arm ramrod straight and vertical, is going to be a bear. No problem, just go as high as you can and gradually build up. Don't rush! Remember that the get-up is an exercise, not a competitive lift. If you are overflowing with testosterone, put it to use on a hard set of swings.

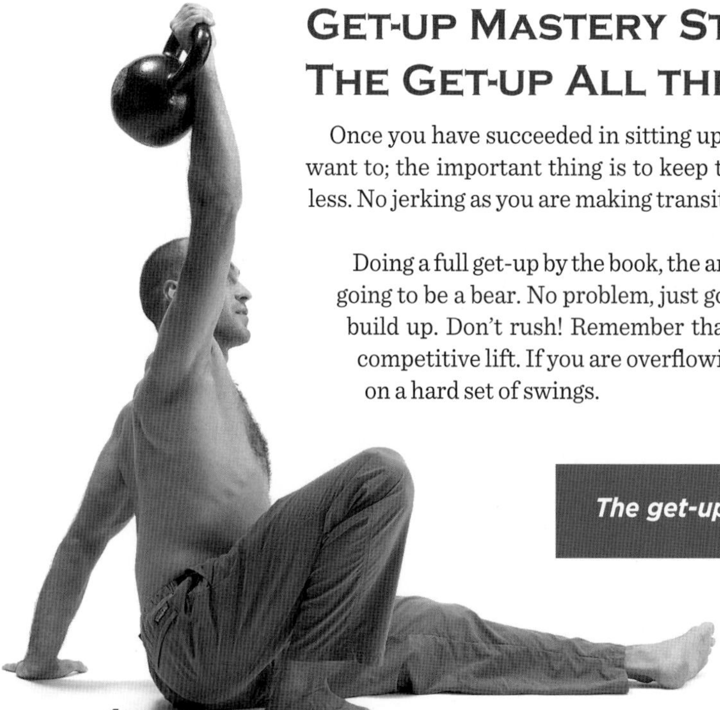

The get-up continued.

4

Lean into the kettlebell on the top for extra stretch. Bring your arm close to your ear (not your ear close to your arm). This may be a good time to revisit the pull-up bar drill by Anthony Diluglio, RKC.

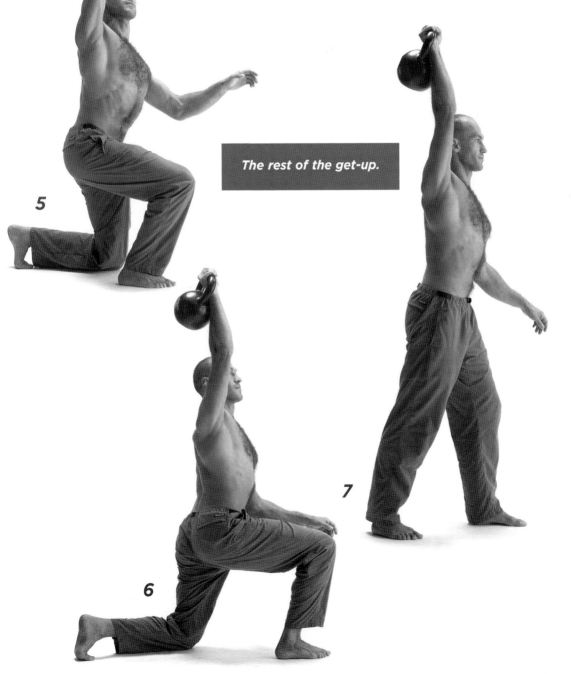

The rest of the get-up.

5

6

7

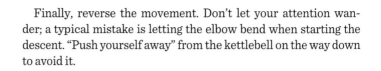

Finally, reverse the movement. Don't let your attention wander; a typical mistake is letting the elbow bend when starting the descent. "Push yourself away" from the kettlebell on the way down to avoid it.

You will not believe how great your shoulders will feel!

8

9

10

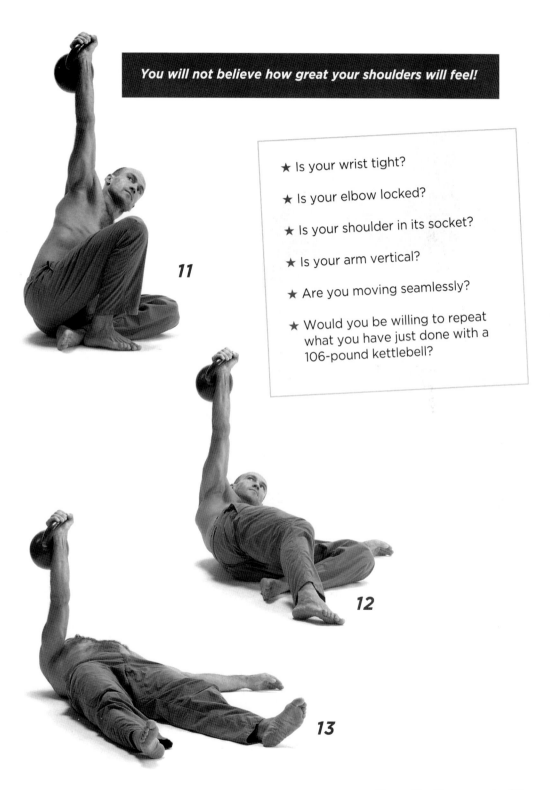

You will not believe how great your shoulders will feel!

★ Is your wrist tight?

★ Is your elbow locked?

★ Is your shoulder in its socket?

★ Is your arm vertical?

★ Are you moving seamlessly?

★ Would you be willing to repeat what you have just done with a 106-pound kettlebell?

11

12

13

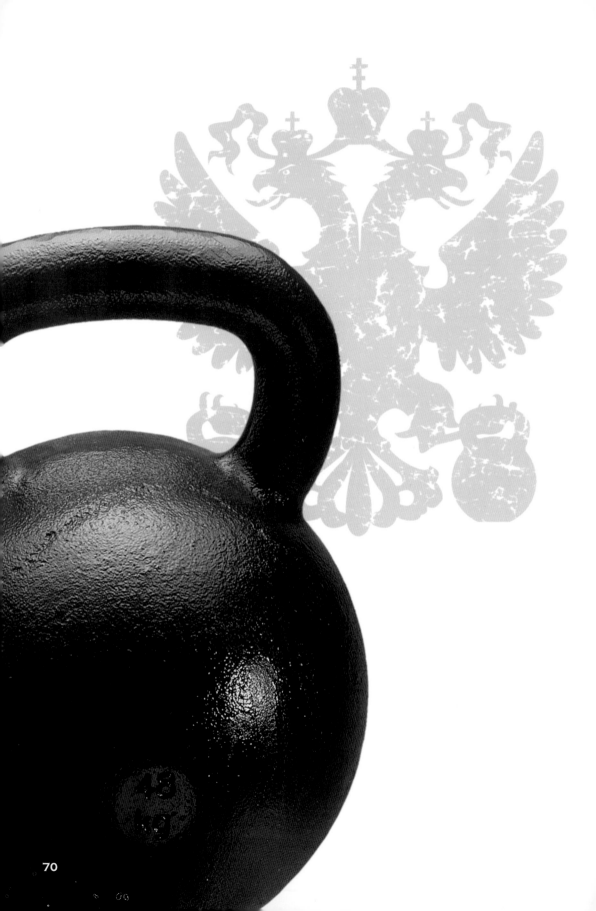

★ ★ ★
THE NEW
RKC PROGRAM
MINIMUM
★ ★ ★

Simple and sinister.

—A U.S. Secret Service Counter Assault Team instructor on the RKC system of training

hen the Communists were plotting their coup on the verge of the XX century, they had a program maximum, for total domination—and a *program minimum*, for the most important and immediate concerns.

The New RKC Program Minimum will deliver

★ The conditioning of a world-class fighter;

★ Rapid fat loss without the dishonor of aerobics;

★ A back of steel;

★ Muscular, flexible, and resilient shoulders;

★ A skill base for the rest of the RKC drills.

Regardless of your goals, a simple routine of swings and get-ups makes a powerful introduction to RKC training. The sales cliché about 80 percent of the business—or more—coming from 20 percent of the clients applies to kettlebell training: these two moves will give you the biggest bang for your kettlebell buck. The swing will take care of your back, legs, heart, and lungs. The get-up will temper flexible and resilient shoulders, ready for exercises and sports skills that traditionally trash them: punching a heavy bag, grappling, heavy pressing and jerking, and so on.

I have experimented with different ways to put swings and get-ups into a routine, but I could not do better than Steve Baccari, RKC. Steve has designed the following "simple and sinister" S&C routine for the grapplers he has been training with.

★ **Twice a week, a hard 12 minutes of the U.S. Department of Energy "Man Maker."**
The Man Maker is a painfully simple workout that was devised and implemented at a federal agency's academy by Green Beret vet Bill Cullen, RKC. Its template is simple: alternate sets of high-rep kettlebell drills—swings in our case—with a few hundred yards of jogging. Do your swings "to a comfortable stop" most of the time and all-out occasionally. Don't run hard; jogging is a form of active recovery. Senior RKC Mike Mahler prefers the jump rope to jogging, another great option.

★ **Twice a week, 5 minutes of continuous get-ups, switching hands every rep.**
Steve's get-up routine gives the shoulders enough time under tension to build serious muscle and keeps them safe by allowing the stabilizers to recover after each rep.

Please note that it is a bad idea to count your get-up reps and especially to try to top them! This exercise requires finesse, not speed. Even if your reps are modest, the shoulder muscles will remain under static tension for a long period of time, exactly what they need to get bigger and stronger. The Brazilian grapplers Baccari has been putting through this routine have developed remarkable shoulders and backs!

Note that there is nothing magical about 5 or 12 minutes. Start with these numbers; you can expand or compress them later. "I picked 5 min because that is the length of a round in both sparing and competition," explains Steve. "As for the 12 min Man Makers, most of the guys had about a 10 min threshold ... so I just bumped it up a step. Most of them are now doing about 15 min."

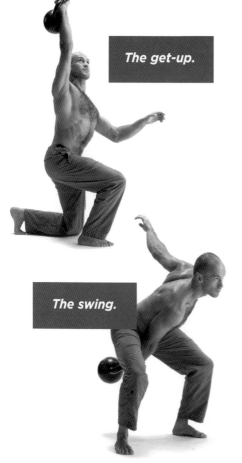

★ ★ ★
THE NEW
RKC PROGRAM
MINIMUM
SUMMARY
★ ★ ★

The get-up.

The swing.

★ Twice a week, alternate sets of swings with easy jogging for recovery for 12 minutes.

★ Do your swings to a comfortable stop. Once you are well conditioned you may go all-out occasionally.

★ "Shake out" the lactic acid and tension from your muscles when jogging. Relax! The purpose of jogging is active recovery, not more conditioning.

★ Twice a week, do get-up singles, switching arms after each rep, for 5 minutes.

★ Focus on perfect technique, not on reps. Don't count your get-up reps, and don't try to top them!

★ Arrange the weekly plan any way you want, e.g., Mon., Thurs.—swings; Tues., Fri.—get-ups or Mon., Thurs.—get-ups; Tues., Sat.—swings. If you want to add an extra swing or get-up day, go ahead—make your day.

★ Start each workout with 10 minutes of face-the-wall squats, halos, and pumps.

★ Unless you are an experienced strength athlete, do no other lifting

THE NEXT STEP

Comrade, once you are rocking on the RKC Program Minimum, start practicing the hard-core exercises from the next chapter—the clean, the press, the snatch—before each workout.

"Practice" the clean, the press, and the snatch; don't "work out"! Set aside 15 minutes before each of your four weekly RKC Program Minimum workouts, right after your face-the wall squats, halos, and pumps. Do a few reps, rest, then do a few more. Go nowhere close to your limit, not even to 50 percent. Kettlebell cleans, presses, and snatches are very demanding in terms of both technique and flexibility, so take your time. Weeks and months if necessary. There is no rush; you are still getting your strength and conditioning from the RKC Program Minimum.

Only when your cleans, presses, and snatches are perfect may you start the RKC Rite of Passage program from the next chapter. The Russian kettlebell does not forgive not paying attention.

Russian kettlebell power to you!

CHAPTER III
THE RKC RITE OF PASSAGE

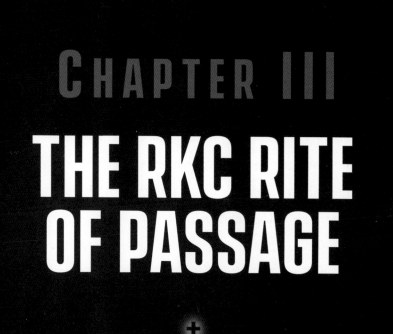

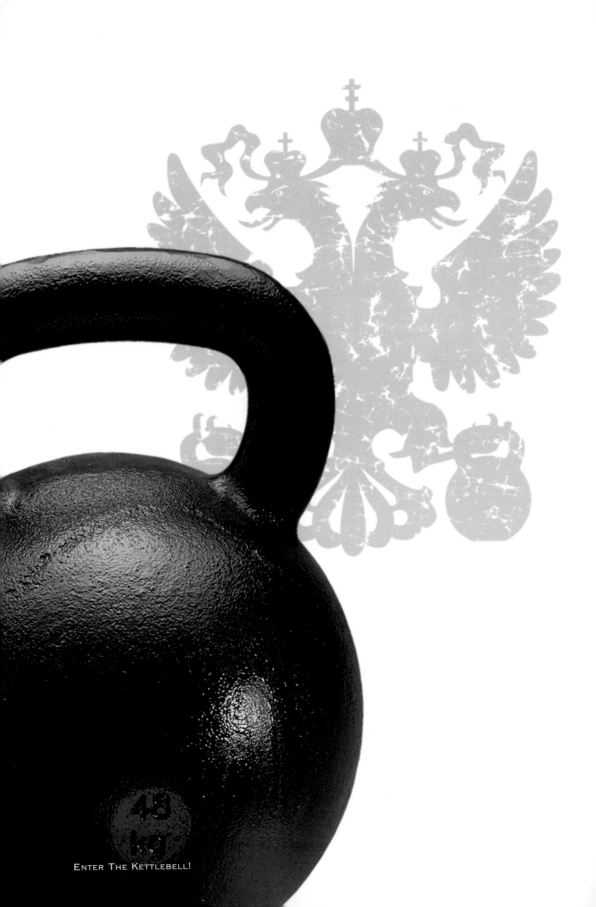

ENTER THE KETTLEBELL!

Chapter 3:

The RKC Rite of Passage

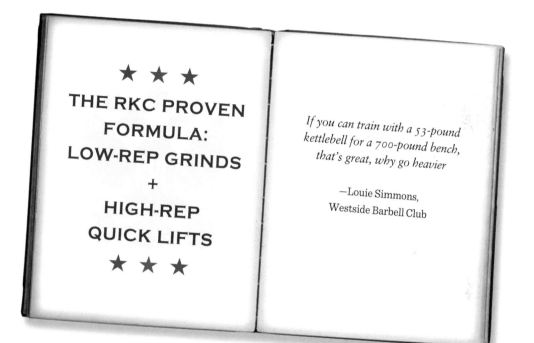

★ ★ ★

THE RKC PROVEN
FORMULA:
LOW-REP GRINDS
+
HIGH-REP
QUICK LIFTS

★ ★ ★

If you can train with a 53-pound kettlebell for a 700-pound bench, that's great, why go heavier

—Louie Simmons,
Westside Barbell Club

The emphasis on brute, low-rep strength differentiates the RKC system. Most S&C methodologies aimed at the military and fighters heavily lean into conditioning while de-emphasizing strength. Probably because it is a lot easier to smoke somebody than to make him strong. RKC practitioners get their share of conditioning, but strength always remains a priority.

Enter "Slow Strength"

Low-rep training, so heavy that the weight barely moves, is the stepchild of the strength-and-conditioning world. Pros and amateurs alike are afraid of low-rep "slow strength" training. After all, doesn't it slow you down? And where is the conditioning?!

Wrong. "Slow strength" happens to be one of the counterintuitive and rarely revealed secrets of Russian athletic might. It is defined as one's ability to exert the greatest force regardless of the time it takes. The guts to grind it through. The powerlifting deadlift and the military press with a heavy kettlebell are classic displays of slow strength. Slow strength is always trained and tested with low repetitions, one to five.

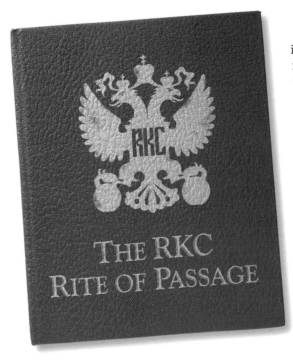

THE RKC RITE OF PASSAGE

"All fighters and coaches understand the importance of roadwork," says Boston boxing coach extraordinaire Steve Baccari, RKC "They understand the importance of working the heavy bag, the hand-pads, and of course, sparring. But what is commonly overlooked, and possibly the most important piece of the strength and conditioning puzzle—is strength training. Or what Pavel refers to as slow strength. What does slow strength do for a boxer? First and foremost, when a fighter has a good strength base, it reduces his chance of injuries. Second, it makes him more resilient in the ring. Finally, strength translates into more power in his punches. After all, power is strength times speed. Most coaches over-emphasize strength endurance. Granted, this is very important, but before you can endure strength, you must first develop it."

Slow, heavy lifts or "grinds," done for one to five reps are one side of the RKC coin. High-rep, quick lifts are the flip side. When we train to "endure strength," we turn everything around: the lifts are quick and the reps are high. Kettlebell swings and snatches done for 10, 100, and even more reps are unbeatable for developing championship conditioning. Countless tough hombres have been humbled by these drills. Fighters, athletes, and special operators have admitted that they were shocked to discover they had met the hardest workout of their lives. Here's how Mike Castrogiovanni, RKC, a strong, tough-as-nails wrestler, describes his first encounter with the Russian kettlebell:

I was visiting with a friend, strength coach Mark Reifkind. He kept on ranting and raving about these things called "Kettlebells." If Mark is ranting about something, you best sit your ass down and take notes. He said, "Look, man, if I told you I had a strength tool that will raise your heart rate over 200BPM you would want to see it, right?"

Now, I've known Rif for quite a while and for him to make a statement like that was pretty absurd, especially since all my kinesiology teachers and textbooks had been telling me that a man of my age should not be able to do so physiologically. After hearing Mark's outlandish claim I decided to pay him a visit to make sure he hadn't killed too many brain cells from all those years of powerlifting and try to bring him back to reality. So, with the intention of proving my old teacher wrong and showing him what a stud I had become, I went to his house.

We went to the garage where I viewed three cannon balls with handles resting on the floor. I thought to myself, "Cannonballs! This guy has lost his marbles." Despite my initial resistance I became very interested as soon as Rif began to demonstrate some of the basic movements. It literally forced my mind to open; I had never seen anything like it nor had I ever been able to conceptualize such a possibility. My experience with explosive movements consisted of the O-lifts which I rarely performed for reps and when I did the reps they certainly were not fluid and continuous. At this point, my interest peaked; but I still felt the skepticism that had been implanted in my mind by the many lectures and late nights of reading. After all, I was on my way to becoming a "Kinesiologist"!

Eventually, my natural child-like curiosity forced my overgrown ego to step down and before I knew it, Mark was teaching me swing techniques, both two and one hand varieties. After Rif felt confident in my ability to perform a safe swing, he introduced the clean and the snatch. It took a little while for me to get the movements down, but eventually I did. The learning process alone elevated my heart rate and breathing. I had begun to think that he might be right and science might be wrong. For the love of God, what was I to do? My whole world was about to collapse before me, in a garage, of all places, at the hands of my old strength coach, of all people, and because of a cannon ball, of all things.

I accepted the inevitable, stood my ground and attacked the bells as if it were my last dance on earth. I remember very little of the workout itself. I know we did swings, cleans, and snatches, and that the workout lasted no more than seven minutes. I remember my heart beating so hard that I could feel it in my pelvic floor, and my heart rate elevated to 221+BPM. [Karvonen formula tables show 195 as "the maximum heart rate" for a 25-year-old.] The thing that stands out most in my mind was my prideful attempts to refrain from vomiting all over Rif's garage and my feeble attempts to act as though I was unaffected by the workout.

Mark Reifkind, RKC, points out another reason kettlebell quick lifts are so valuable: they teach the natural athletic rhythm of tension and relaxation. A former powerlifter and powerlifting coach, Rif could not help noticing how stiff and tight Comrades who do nothing but slow, heavy grinds get.

Tension and relaxation are the two sides of the performance coin. An always-tight powerlifter can hardly move. An always-loose yoga practitioner is weak. A karate master, who moves like lightning and then freezes for a split second to put all of his mass behind the punch and then recoil with relaxed quickness like a snake's tongue, has both. In the words of the late Okinawan karate master Chozo Nakama, this is "relaxed tension."

Like hard-style karate punches, RKC kettlebell swings and snatches rely on a rapid-fire sequence of high tension and relaxation. "Tense-loose-tense-loose." A killer one-two combination for the gym and the ring.

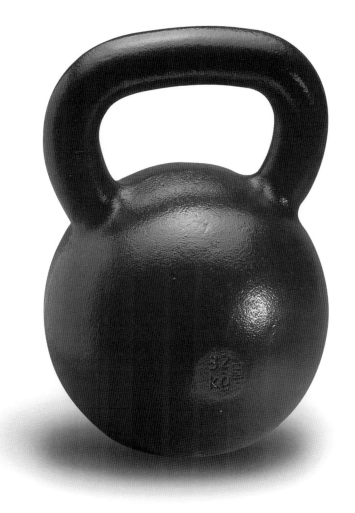

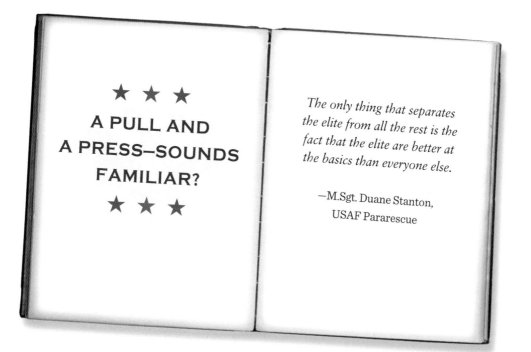

★ ★ ★

A PULL AND A PRESS—SOUNDS FAMILIAR?

★ ★ ★

The only thing that separates the elite from all the rest is the fact that the elite are better at the basics than everyone else.

—M.Sgt. Duane Stanton,
USAF Pararescue

P avel," wrote Texas powerlifter Phil Workman, RKC. "I have been training a friend of mine using the PTP [the ultra-abbreviated routine from *Power to the People!*] for the deadlift and he has made great progress (315 dead to 450 in about a year). Now he wants to do kettlebells but would like to use a PTP format. Is there any workout for the kettlebells that would be close to the PTP?"

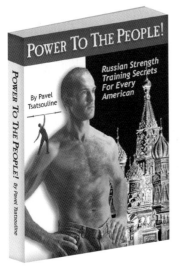

Enter the Kettlebell focuses on doing fewer things better. I have ruthlessly reduced the number of exercises, even if they were favorites of mine. (See you later, windmill!) You will structure your training around the familiar *Power to the People!* foundation of one overhead press and one full-body pull. Note that this is what the RKC Program Minimum is made up of. The swing is a "big" pull, and the get-up can be classified as a static press.

An ultra-abbreviated program consisting of a pull and a press has the power to spectacularly fill most Comrades' strength needs. For a couple of years I have been following the posts of Eddie "the Green Ghost" Kowacz on the RussianKettlebell.com forum. Eddie is a USMC and SWAT veteran, a defensive tactics instructor, and a World Martial Arts Hall of Fame Instructor of the Year.

"When my father saw my full set of KBs," Eddie wrote me, "he knew what they were right away. He spent time in Russia during WW2 and remembers the Russian soldiers swinging them in the sub-zero cold of Kolyma. He saw me do some and was pleased by what he saw and smiled so I must thank you for that."

This hard man's training has been narrowly focused on military presses with two kettlebells and variations of a "big pull": dead lifts and kettlebell swings and snatches. Details vary—for instance, Eddie might do hang snatches and swings with rubber bands attached to the kettlebells, but the essence of the Green Ghost's training has remained the same: a big pull plus an overhead press.

Now why a pull rather than a squat? Big pulls—kettlebell swings and snatches, barbell dead lifts, Olympic pulls—will not replace squats if you are after huge legs or you compete in PL or WL. But if you are not, they rule.

Eddie "the Green Ghost" pulls rather than squats because his knees are "plastic," as he puts it. Unlike squats, even very heavy pulls **rarely irritate the knees**.

Ken Shamrock of UFC fame pulls rather than squats because a fighter has no need for heavier legs. Pulls **strengthen the legs and hips without overdeveloping them**. Chafing is no fun. And for some comrades, for instance special operators and infantrymen, bloody thighs are simply unacceptable. I was walking in the officers' quarters with a Marine friend who had just returned from a tour in Fallujah. We had just worked out and had our shorts on. A passing-by jarhead buddy of his joked, "Are those your legs, or are you riding a chicken?!" Fighting men ride chickens (they don't eat them). Got a problem with that?

As Randall Strossen, PhD, put it, to a man of strength a muscular back is what big arms are to a bodybuilder. Pulls **build backs**.

For reasons listed in the FAQ chapter, kettlebell pulls **dramatically reduce your chances of a back injury**.

"Kettlebell swings work the abs well," observed famous powerlifting coach Louie Simmons. At least in experienced lifters—who employ a heavy kettlebell, crisp technique, and forceful breathing.

Dr. Fred "Squat" Hatfield stated, "The best grip exercises are always going to be pulling at heavy weights ballistically." Kettlebell pulls **forge a vice grip**.

"Coach, I just don't get tired!" This is music to the ears of Chris Holder, RKC, strength coach for the teams at Cal Poly San Luis Obispo. Repetition kettlebell swings and snatches **develop championship conditioning and burn fat without the dishonor of aerobics**.

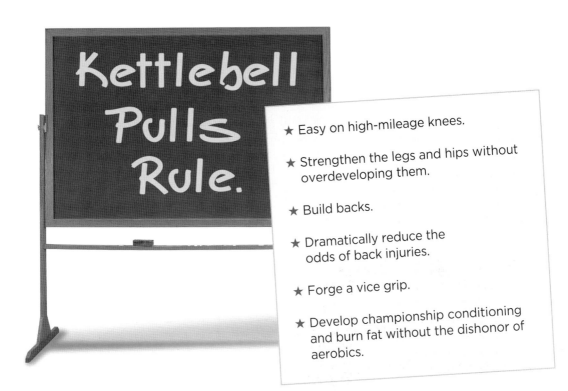

Kettlebell Pulls Rule.

★ Easy on high-mileage knees.

★ Strengthen the legs and hips without overdeveloping them.

★ Build backs.

★ Dramatically reduce the odds of back injuries.

★ Forge a vice grip.

★ Develop championship conditioning and burn fat without the dishonor of aerobics.

Do not interpret the above as a statement that squats hurt your knees. Contrary to the conventional wisdom, properly done squats are great for the knees. "Does this dress make my butt look big?" a woman asks her husband. "No, honey, your butt makes your butt look big." On the same note, Dan John has nailed the truth about squatting: "Squatting does not hurt your knees, the way YOU squat hurts your knees."

Squat—if you are taught how to do it properly and if it is consistent with your goals. We teach the front squat at the RKC instructor certification course. But the foundation of the RKC system will always be the Big Pull.

As for presses, militaries and other overheads, they fill in the small gaps in your armor left by the pulls' blanket bombing. It is obvious that overhead presses strengthen the shoulders, the upper back, and the arms. What is less obvious is their effect on the lats—when you press the RKC way. One of my students, Justin Qualler, RKC, accidentally worked up to a one-arm chin by focusing on pulling his kettlebell military press negatives with his lat!

"After years of dreaming—my eighth grade gym teacher said he'd pay 100 bucks to anyone who could do a one-arm pull-up—and relatively little doing, I stumbled upon, quite accidentally, the side road to the one-arm pullup," wrote Justin in his article for RussianKettlebell.com. "You can bet that I used every tension technique that Pavel's books talk about, including the anal lock, power breathing, ab and glute flexion, and the crush grip. Learn the techniques well. . . . The unexpected exercise that helped me on the OAP side road was the military press. . . . I was pulling hard with my lat on the negative of every rep. Actively pulling down with your lat will groove a motion strikingly similar to the OAP. . . . Remember: you must pull like hell with your lat when the weight is descending!

There's no magic formula, but at some point you'll feel very comfortable and strong when you are pulling the weight down.... It took me a few months. Then one day I tried an OAP and was surprised that I could actually pull myself up—but I couldn't do a complete rep. Remember, I had not been training pullups at all during this time."

A short stretch of pull-up practice and Justin bagged his OAP. Don't hold your breath hoping to repeat Justin's feat, but you will definitely build strong lats if you press the Party way.

As soon as you start pressing heavy, you will be pleasantly surprised at the powerful effect this drill has on your abs and obliques. "Trust me, a forty-five minute workout of Military Presses will work the abdominal muscles as well as any machine advertised on late night television," assures Dan John, a thrower and weightlifter with a cult-like following.

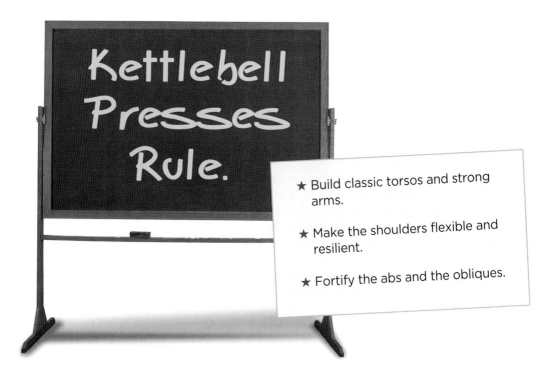

Kettlebell Presses Rule.

★ Build classic torsos and strong arms.

★ Make the shoulders flexible and resilient.

★ Fortify the abs and the obliques.

Following is an ambitious yet realistic set of goals for a regular guy aspiring to be a hard guy:

★ The U.S. Secret Service 10-minute snatch with a 24-kilogram kettlebell—200 reps.

★ The clean-and-press with the kettlebell closest to half your bodyweight—1 rep with each arm.

The Secret Service snatch, explained further on in the book, will build a fighting man's spirit and conditioning, melt the fat without the dishonor of aerobics, develop hard-driving hip power for unstoppable tackles and hard hits, and make other men take notice when you shake hands.

The heavy kettlebell press builds an upper body ready to take and dish out punishment. In some parts of Russia, pressing a two-pood is a rite of passage from boy to man. As it should be.

Here is what Comrades ladies should shoot for:

★ The USSS 10-minute snatch with a 12-kilogram kettlebell—200 reps.

★ The C&P with the kettlebell closest to a quarter of your bodyweight—
1 rep with each arm.

It may take you a year, two, or more to bring your strength and conditioning up to this level; take your time. When you make these goals, your brute strength, explosive power, and conditioning will impress, you will have muscles in all the right places and no body fat to speak of. You will be strong enough to be accepted as a man among men.

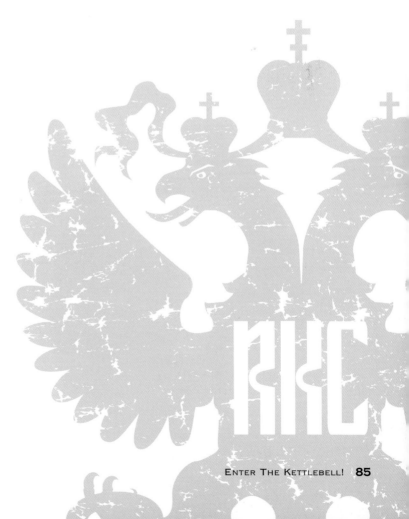

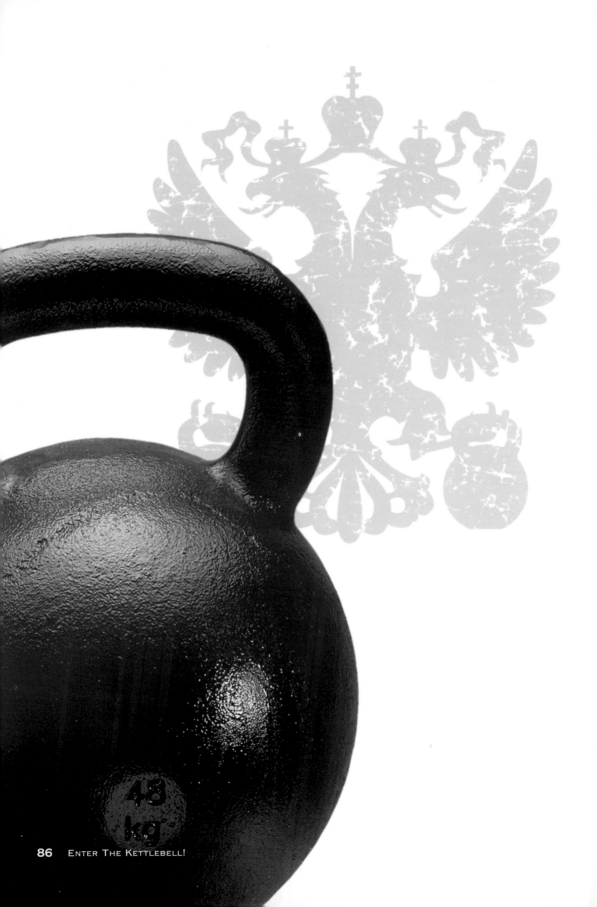

★ ★ ★
THE
CLEAN
–CRISP
LIKE A PUNCH
★ ★ ★

The swinging of kettlebells requires a strong forearm and wrist

—George "the Russian Lion" Hackenschmidt

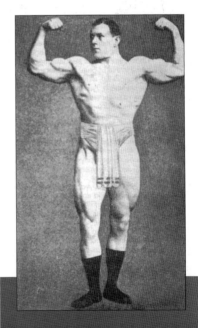

George "the Russian Lion" Hackenschmidt

The clean draws its name from the requirement to bring the weight from the ground to your shoulders in one "clean" movement. In the RKC system of training, single kettlebell cleans are not used on their own—too easy—but in a pair with presses. Except when you are learning to clean.

The kettlebell clean technique is very different from the one employed by Olympic lifters. The biggest differences are not shrugging the shoulders, keeping the elbows in, and not puffing out the chest.

Note that while the clean is one of the easiest exercises one can do with a given size of kettlebell, it is one of the more difficult ones to do right—without banging your forearm or yanking your elbow. So take your time practicing, just a few reps every day rather than a lot in one shot. The cleaner your clean, the bigger your press.

Task: Clean

Condition:
Pick up a kettlebell, swing it back between your legs as if for a swing, and bring it to the rack in one smooth movement. Then drop the kettlebell back between your legs and repeat the drill for reps.

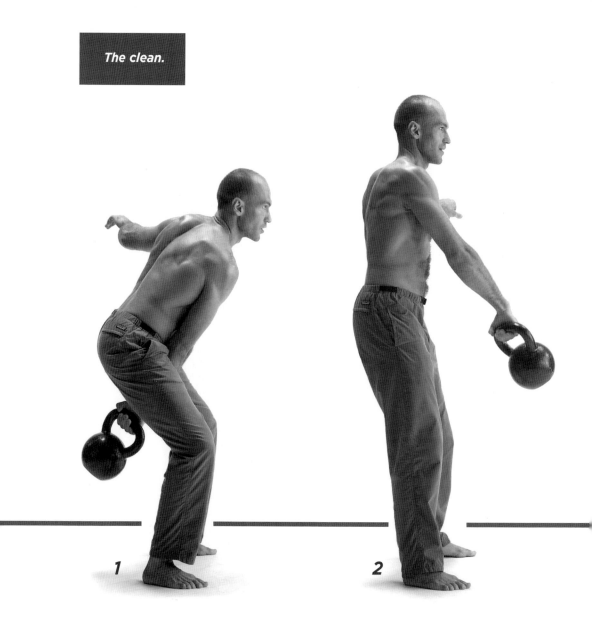

The clean.

1

2

Standard:

1. All of the points that apply to the swing, minus the straight-arm requirement on the top.
2. Don't dip your knees when racking the kettlebell.
3. The kettlebell, the elbow, and the torso must "become one" on the top of the clean.

   The shoulders must be pressed down.
4. The arms must stay loose, and the hips must do all the work.
5. The kettlebell must travel the shortest distance possible.
6. Unacceptable: scooping; banging the forearms; stressing the back, elbows, wrists, or shoulders. Ladies should not hit their breasts with their arms or the kettlebells for health reasons.

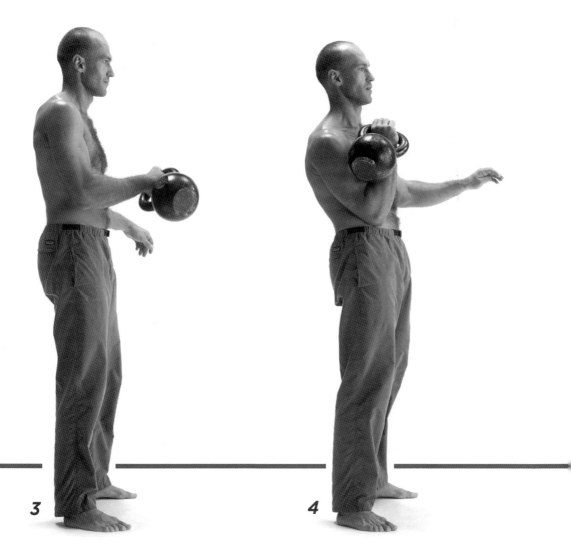

3

4

Clean Mastery Step #1: the Grip

Having studied boxing greats, Bruce Lee once commented, "There are no wrists in boxing.... The forearm and the fist should be used as one solid piece, like a club with a knot on the end of it. The fist should be kept on a straight line with the forearm and there should be no bending of the wrist in any direction." Ditto with the kettlebell lifts. A limp wrist bent back is a guarantee of weakness and injuries.

There is a difference between the grip for the get-up and other slow lifts or "grinds"—and the grip for the clean and the quick lifts. The ballistics do not require you to crush the handle; you can even keep your hand open and wiggle the fingers. Just don't let your wrist cave in.

Pick your kettlebell up with two hands. Spear one hand through the handle while holding up the ball with the other. Push deeper. Wiggle your hand around to find a comfortable spot. Keep adjusting until the handle rests on the very heel of your palm, almost sliding down onto your forearm.

Let go with the supporting hand and let the ball rest on the outside of your forearm. Wiggle your fingers some more to relieve the pressure on the forearm and to become "one with the kettlebell." You should feel more weight on your forearm than on your palm.

When the kettlebell is in motion don't grip it, just hook the handle with your fingers.

Pick up the kettlebell with two hands, then let go with one.

1

2

Clean Mastery Step #2: the Rack

Senior RKC Rob Lawrence has dramatically accelerated our students' clean mastery by proposing to study the clean in reverse: the rack, the drop, the clean proper. If your weightlifting is not up to snuff, "the rack" refers to holding a weight on your chest.

Cheat curl a kettlebell with two hands. Adjust your grip and let go with the assisting hand. Move around to find the sweet spot where you become "one with the kettlebell."

A girevik's posture is the opposite of a strutting bodybuilder's. The shoulders are stretched down, the chest is not puffed out, the shoulder blades are spread out like a fighter's, the elbows are tightly pressed against the body (no imaginary lats, Comrade!), and the hips are slightly pushed forward. Ori Hofmekler, Israeli spec ops vet and the author of *The Warrior Diet*, calls this alignment "the warrior posture."

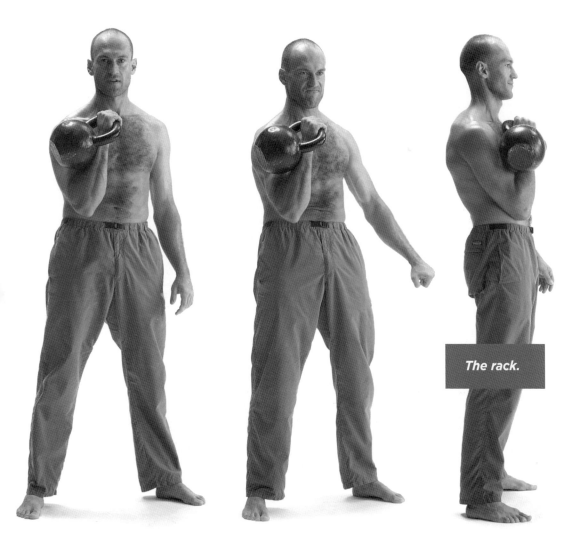

The rack.

Do not support the kettlebell by shrugging your shoulder or pushing up with your arm. Relax your shoulder girdle and let the weight of the kettlebell pass directly to your rib cage, stomach, and hips. Your elbow must go as low as possible.

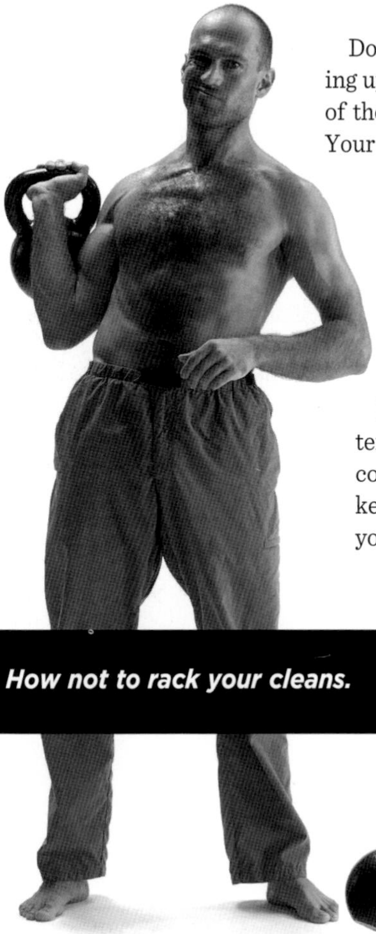

It is important to keep some tension in your glutes—pinch a coin—to protect your back. Also keep some braced tension in your abs.

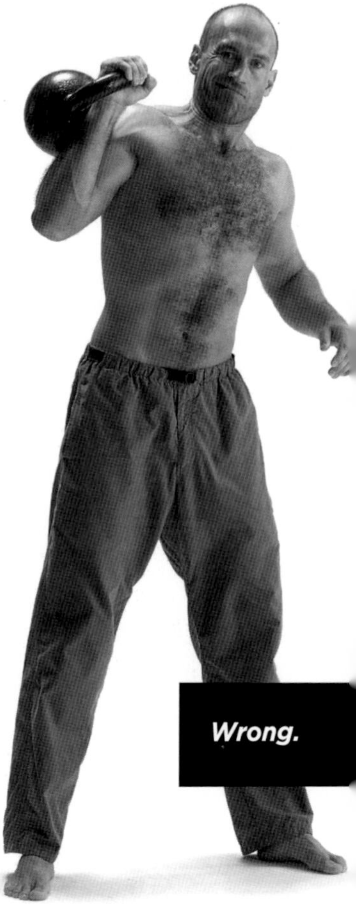

How not to rack your cleans.

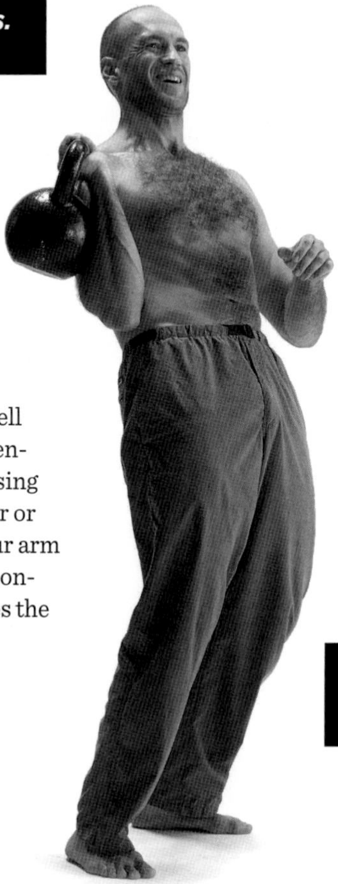

Wrong.

Unlike a dumbbell, a kettlebell must be racked close to your centerline. Imagine that you are using your elbow to protect your liver or spleen from a punch. Press your arm against your ribs. An arm "disconnected" from the body punishes the shoulder.

Wrong.

The last point does not apply to ladies. For health reasons, it is not advisable that women apply pressure to their breasts with kettlebells, upper arms, or forearms. Which is why they must resort to a more awkward, wider position with the forearm and the kettlebell outside their breasts. Be careful not to end up in what arm-wrestlers call "the broken-arm position"—the fist heading sideways or backward while the elbow is staying in. A mental experiment should convince you that this will do the inside of your elbow no good.

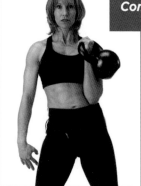

Comrades ladies must finish their cleans more to the side.

Regardless of your gender, the kettlebell should fit comfortably into the "triangle" of your elbow. If it does not, the top of your forearm will experience a lot of pressure from the ball.

Once you have become one with the kettlebell, hold the rack until fatigue forces you to put the kettlebell down—with two hands, please. Keep your glutes slightly tensed, and don't forget to breathe. Standing or walking with a kettlebell racked will force your traps to relax—it is "forced relaxation"—and help you find a comfortable rack.

Don't proceed to the next step until your rack is perfect!

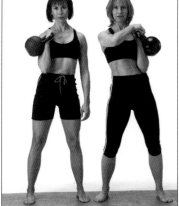

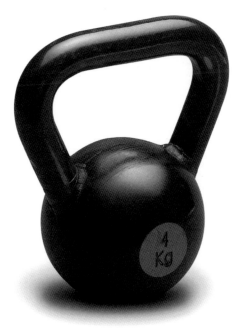

CLEAN MASTERY STEP #3: THE DROP

When the kettlebell is dropped from the rack back between the legs, it must be literally dropped with a totally loose arm. The arm must stay relaxed and straighten out completely on the bottom of the drop. The shock is then absorbed by the hips.

Negative curling the bell invites elbow problems. Arm tension is a sign of fear. You are afraid of getting injured by the momentum of the kettlebell. But, as often is the case, fear is a self-fulfilling prophecy. Here is how to build your confidence and a relaxed drop:

Practice on a surface where you can safely throw the kettlebell. Start with the kettlebell in the rack. Push your butt back, relax your arm, and turn your thumb slightly down as if you are pouring vodka. The kettlebell will roll off your forearm.

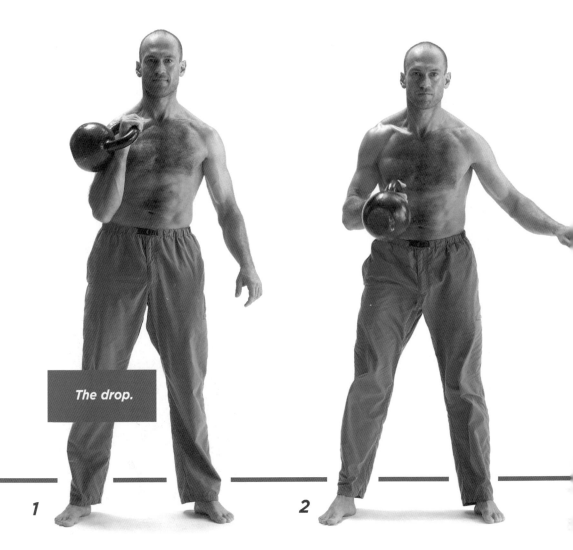

The drop.

1   2

Don't throw the kettlebell forward; keep it as close to your body as possible!

Don't grip the handle; hook it loosely with your fingers.

Don't let your elbow flare; it must move toward the centerline.

Throw the kettlebell behind you between your legs—not straight down. Just like the hike pass from football. The closer your forearm is to your groin, the better. The tighter the arc, the better. Taming the arc is a very important concept in kettlebell quick lifts.

Your fist keeps turning more and more until your thumb is pointing almost straight down at the very bottom. Note that the turn of the fist must be seamless, like a kung fu block. A jerky transition is not welcomed by your elbow.

Your arm should completely—and loosely!—straighten out at the time the kettlebell is behind you. Now you should look like a witch riding a broomstick—your forearm. Your weight must be on your heels, and you must look straight ahead. You should feel your hips loading but not your back. This is the moment to release your kettlebell. Yes, just let it rip behind you.

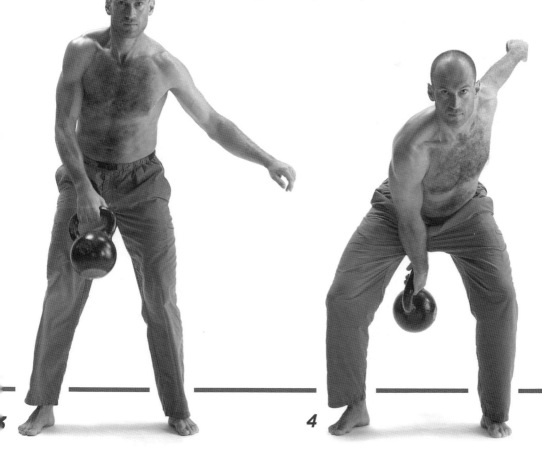

3

4

Keep practicing, and don't attempt cleans until your drop is loose as a whip.

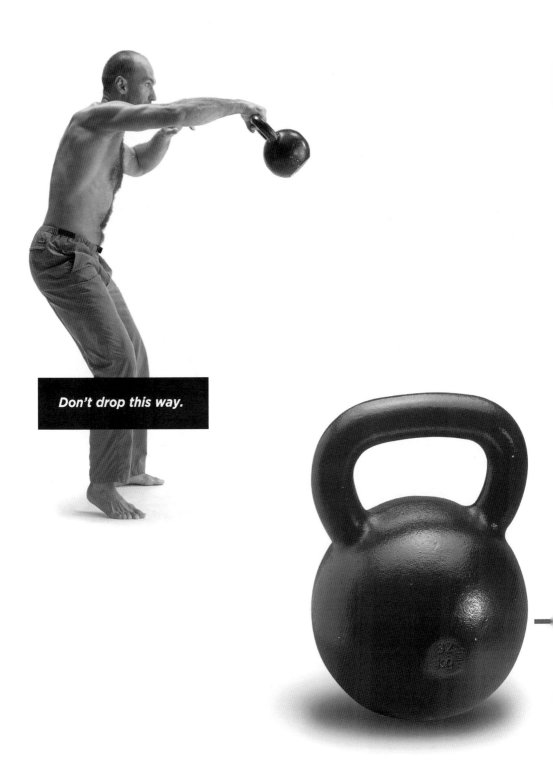

Don't drop this way.

Clean Mastery Step #4: the Clean Proper

When you have achieved a relaxed drop, don't release the kettlebell on the bottom of the drop, but snap your hips and let the kettlebell come up, retracing its drop trajectory.

As simple as that. If you give it any more thought, you are likely to make a series of mistakes: pulling with the arm rather than the hips, banging your forearm, and so on. Just retrace the drop.

Spear your hand through the handle as the bell is coming home, to make sure the weight will rest as low on your palm as possible.

Let the kettlebell roll around your forearm rather than flip over your fist.

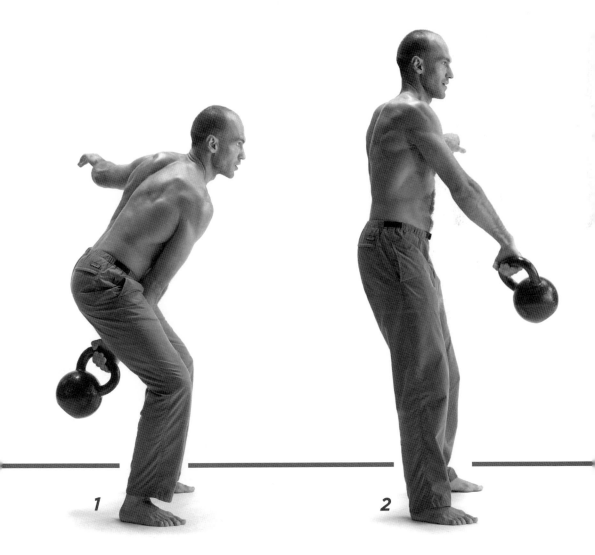

1   2

Senior RKC Mike Mahler compares the final stage of the clean to an uppercut: "Focus on getting your hand around the bell rather than letting the bell flip over and smack you. As the bell passes waist level, imagine that you are doing an uppercut and get your hand around the bell. Make a fist at the top to get the bell in line with you."

Catch the kettlebell as low as possible; it helps to visualize that you are cleaning to your waist rather than your shoulder.

Tense your glutes and brace your abs—don't suck them in, but wall them up as you would for a punch—to absorb the impact. Don't rebend your knees.

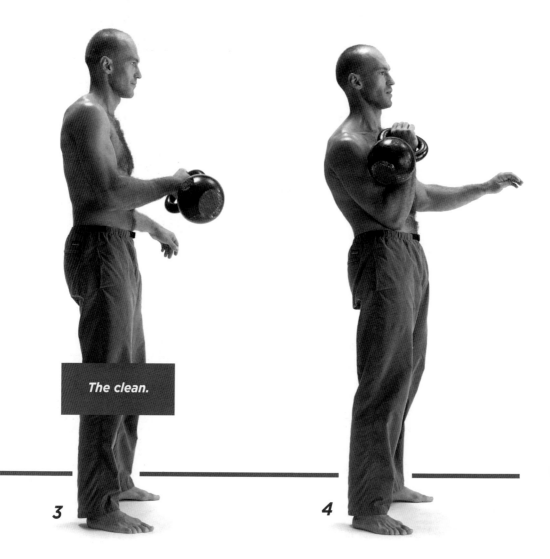

The clean.

3

4

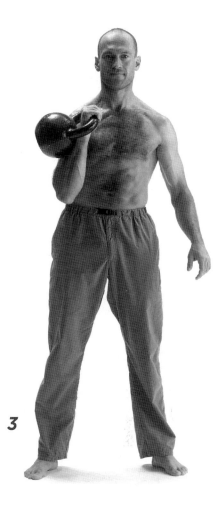

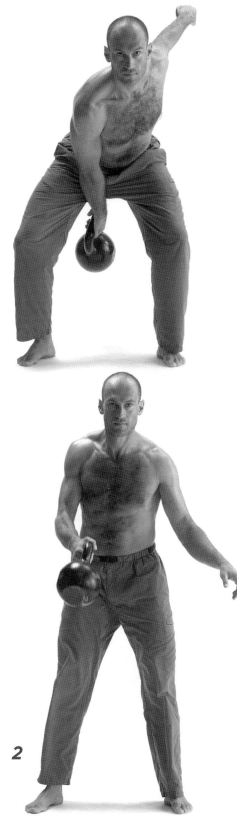

"Focus on getting your hand around the bell rather than letting the bell flip over and smack you. As the bell passes waist level, imagine that you are doing an uppercut and get your hand around the bell. Make a fist at the top to get the bell in line with you."

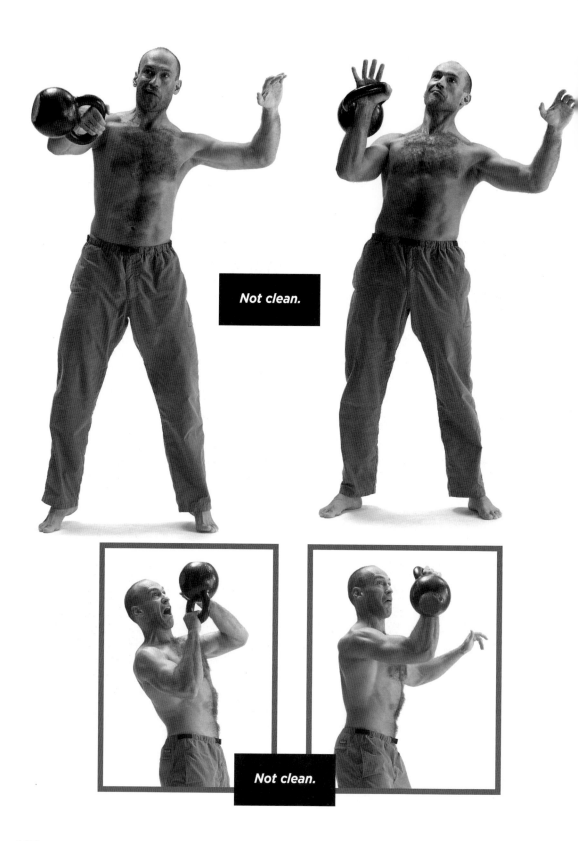

Not clean.

Not clean.

As with the squat, the wall will help you with your clean technique. Do a few cleans with the side of your foot, on the working side, touching or almost touching a wall. This will force you not to clean to the "broken-arm position." Keep your other hand up to block the kettlebell should it bounce off the wall!

Likewise, facing the wall and cleaning will teach you to tame the arc. Keep your guard up!

You must realize now that the clean, although a basic move, is not so simple to master. I will say it again: take your time with it and never make many attempts per session. It is boring, but tell someone who cares.

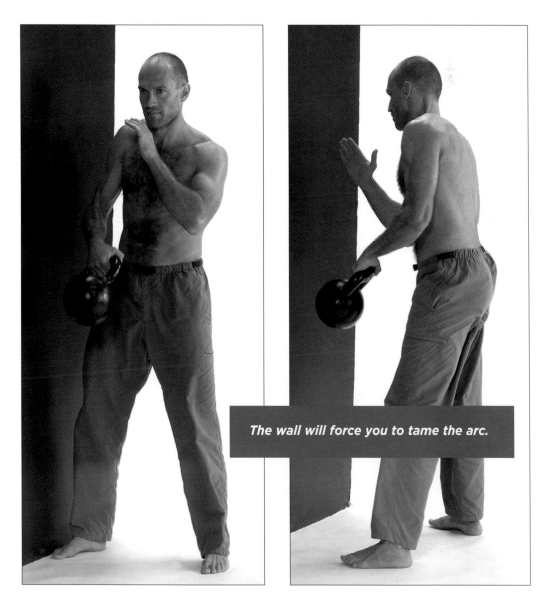

The wall will force you to tame the arc.

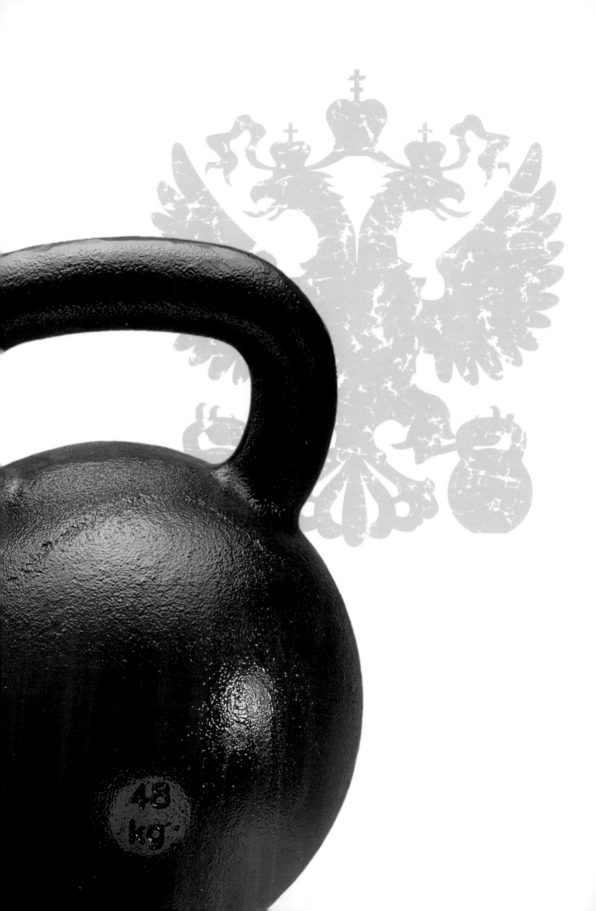

★ ★ ★

THE PRESS
—FOR A
CLASSIC
TORSO

★ ★ ★

I was still a boy but pressed kettlebells with ease and felt like a man.
Even when I fell for the barbell I still loved training with kettlebells.

—Leonid Zhabotinskiy, two-time Olympic weightlifting champion

It is no coincidence that since overhead presses have fallen out of favor, manly Farnese Hercules torsos with powerful shoulders and midsections have given way to small, feminine waists and large pecs. What a shame, because if you work your overhead presses hard, you will hardly need to do anything else for your upper body.

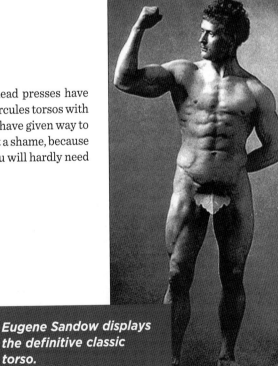

Eugene Sandow displays the definitive classic torso.

TASK: CLEAN AND MILITARY PRESS

Condition:

Clean a kettlebell and press it strictly overhead to lockout.

Standard:
1. Pause motionless, with the kettlebell racked long enough to make sure you will not be using the momentum generated by the clean, for the press.
2. Press with your knees locked and with a minimal back and/or side bend.
3. Keep your whole body tight, especially the midsection, glutes, and quads.
4. Keep your pressing shoulder down.
5. Lock out your elbow completely and pause motionless.

Caution: The following high-tension and power-breathing techniques are not appropriate for Comrades with heart problems or high blood pressure!

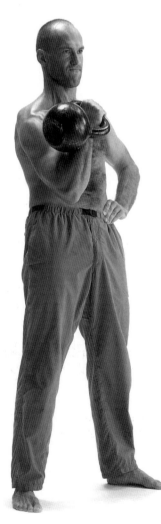

PRESS MASTERY STEP #1: THE LOADED CLEAN

Your press is only as good as your clean. Watch a newbie clean and press a kettlebell. The clean will rock him off balance, almost making him stagger backward. He will then put up a shaky press, his feet and waist wiggling all over the place.

Now watch an expert do the same thing. The kettlebell pro is the indisputable master of the forces he generates. The heavy kettlebell will not push him around. Instead, the kinetic energy will do something very cool. It will not dissipate back over his shoulder but rather go straight down his body into his feet. Every muscle will tense, and his whole body will compress like a spring. After a legal pause, the stored energy will rebound explosively from the feet in a crisp display of strength as he presses the kettlebell.

An experienced girevik is playing a game of "force pool," expertly rebounding the force generated by the clean from the ground. When—or if—you master this skill you will wield awesome pressing power.

The loaded clean.

As you rack your clean, maximally tighten your whole body on impact: your feet, your quads, your glutes, your abs, your lats. It is not just about shock absorption; bracing for the weight will make the kettlebell feel like a toy in your hand, and your muscles will be powerfully loaded for action.

According to Russian sports scientist Professor Yuri Verkhoshansky, isometrically tensing your muscles before a dynamic contraction can improve your performance by up to 20 percent! A good arm-wrestler loads all his muscles with high-strung tension before the ref yells "Go!" A great arm-wrestler will load even before he grips up with his opponent. And an amateur who waits for the referee's command to pull before turning on his biceps finds himself pinned without knowing what has hit him. So brace yourself while the bell is still in the air, not when it hits you. Houdini could take anyone's punch if he was prepared for it. He died after he got struck without warning.

Don't dip your knees when racking your clean! If you have read *The Russian Kettlebell Challenge*, you must remember that I used to recommend dipping your knees. Not any more. I have found that gireviks who dip lose the tightness required for a heavy press. I never stop polishing my training system, which is why you will find a few inconsistencies between *The Russian Kettlebell Challenge* and *Enter the Kettlebell!* The latter book takes precedence. At the RKC we never rest.

Note that although your presses will not be at their strongest without a strong clean, you can start practicing presses before total clean mastery. Clean the kettlebell with the two-handed pistol grip, then release one hand for the press. Following the press, you may drop the kettlebell from the chest with two hands as well.

PRESS MASTERY STEP #2:
PUSH YOURSELF AWAY FROM THE KETTLEBELL

To get the most out of your press while putting the least amount of stress on your shoulder, you must start the lift with your shoulder maximally pressed down—the opposite of a shrug—and your elbow pushed as low as it can go. At the same time, pull the elbow slightly inward toward your belly button. It will feel like you are stretching the "bow" of your deltoid.

Keeping that shoulder down throughout the press will make the press stronger and safer, but it is not an easy skill to develop. Here is cool drill that will help you master it and teach you to stay tight too.

Stand inside a doorway, raise both arms overhead, and place your hands on the supporting beam as if you are military pressing it. Ideally, your hands should be slightly above your head. Unless you play for the NBA, you will need a sturdy box to stand on.

Grip the ground with your toes. Flex your quads and pull up your kneecaps. Cramp your glutes. Brace your abs for a punch (don't suck them in). Breathe shallowly throughout the exercise, but without relaxing your abs. As some karatekas say, "Breathe behind the shield."

Now push up against the top of the doorway with moderate effort. Note what it feels like. Relax. After a brief rest, gather the tension in your body from your feet up, and this time, instead of pushing up, focus on pushing yourself away from the doorway down into the ground. Try to leave foot imprints in the carpet. Note that your knees must remain locked, and your back must be braced with a muscular corset.

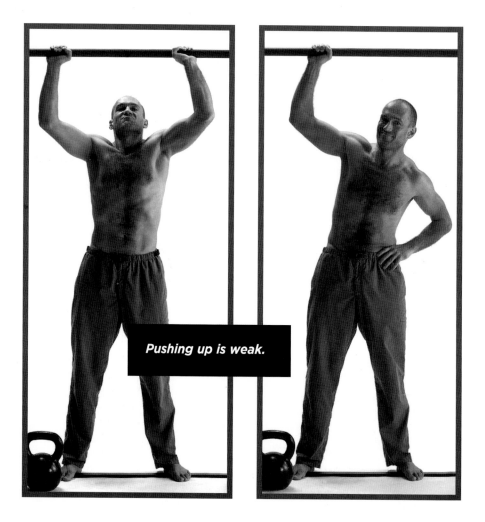

Pushing up is weak.

Something curious will happen: You will feel that your tense body has compacted and gotten shorter. Your shoulders have been sucked into their sockets and feel great. And your pressing power has gone way up!

Remember this feeling of tightness and pushing yourself away when you are pressing a live weight. Greater strength and shoulder resilience will be your rewards.

Note that you must stay cool for this to work. When you doubt your strength and panic, you can't help thinking of lifting the kettlebell instead of pushing yourself away from it. Your shoulder will come up, and the kettlebell with it. But only for a couple of inches. And then it will die. Patience and confidence are prerequisites to great strength.

Now try the same isometric press with one arm. You will notice that you need to tense your obliques more. You will also observe that you will have to play with your body position to find a strong connection between your hand and your feet.

Scan your body for any slack areas that Steve Baccari, RKC, appropriately calls "leakages." Plug them with tension. Wedge yourself between the top of the doorway and the floor. Locked. Rooted. Remember that feeling for your kettlebell press.

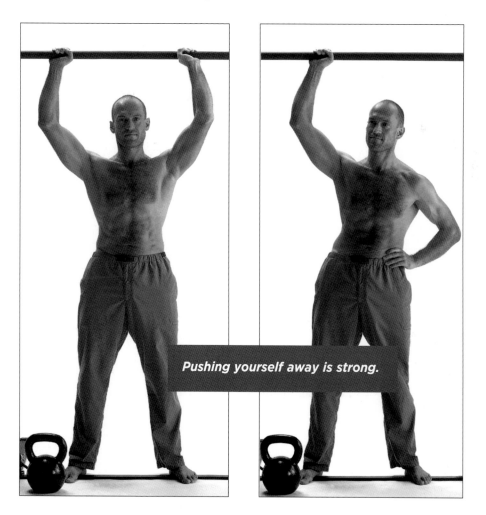

Pushing yourself away is strong.

PRESS MASTERY STEP #3: THE GROOVE

Do not press the bell straight up; your delts will have no leverage. The groove of the kettlebell military press is similar to that of the Arnold press: Start with your palm in the semicurl position, and turn it forward as you press. Press the bell somewhat outward rather than straight up, and be sure to keep your forearm vertical at all times. Unlike the Arnold press, the Russian military press demands that you lock your elbow at the top.

Visualize pushing outward with your elbow—sort of a "lateral raise meets the reverse pec deck"—while keeping your forearm vertical rather than angled toward your head. It is elementary mechanics, Watson: you will never press a heavy weight overhead unless you keep the forearm vertical. Consider almost overdoing it the other way: push the weight away from your body almost to the point where it falls sideways. You will recruit more muscles in the effort—even your biceps. The kettlebell's unique design enables you to push out with your forearm against the "ball" of the kettlebell. This effectively "shortens" your forearm, improving your leverage.

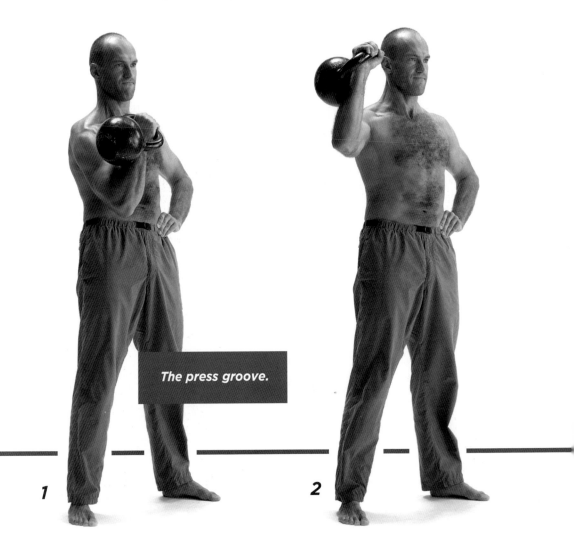

The press groove.

1

2

Squeeze the girya as you press it, and remember to keep your wrist tight. Make sure that the bell's handle rests on the meaty spot at the very base of your palm on the little finger side.

Keep your shoulder pressed down as much as possible throughout the press. Remember to visualize that you are pushing yourself away from the weight rather than pressing it up.

Finish the lift slow and tight, and lock out the elbow firmly. Do not even bother listening to the big sissies who tell you never to lock your joints. The joints need strengthening as much as the muscles do, and locking out is the way to do it. Flexibility is another issue. Look at the photos and observe that the hip is kicked over to the side slightly in order to get positioned straight under the bell. It is all about physics. A heavy kettlebell's plumb line must be projected over your feet if you do not feel like toppling over.

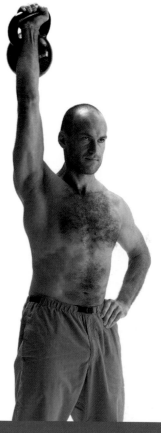

Push your forearm against the ball for better leverage.

3

4

"Heavy" is relative, of course—relative to your body weight rather than your strength. RKCs Bud Jeffries and Donnie Thompson, who weigh a good deal over 300, have no problem pressing the 106-pound Beast standing at attention. On the other hand, 170-pound Senior RKC Steve Cotter has plenty of strength to strictly press the Beast, but not enough body mass to anchor himself to do it standing ramrod straight. Newton's fault.

Realize that displacing the hips sideways does not give you an excuse to lean back, which could be bad news for some backs. An intense ab and glute contraction will help you to avoid leaning back, no matter how heavy the weight is.

Look straight ahead when pressing. Looking up, while making your triceps and chest stronger, tempts you to lean back. Also, as Russian weight lifters used to say, pressing overhead while looking up may "bite the neck," in other words, kink it. So save this trick until you are one bad hombre.

PRESS MASTERY STEP #4:
USE THE BREATH TO MAINTAIN TENSION

You should have taken a normal breath before you even cleaned the weight. When you are pressing, hold your breath or breathe shallowly while keeping your abs hard. As Uechi-ryu karate practitioners say, "Breathe behind the shield"—a great expression to describe this type of breathing.

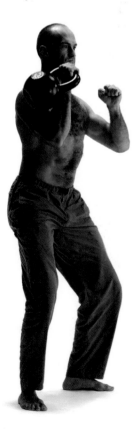

If you are a student of *Power to the People!* or *The Naked Warrior*, you may employ various "power breathing" techniques. The important thing about your breathing is that it does not make you lose tension! When you lose tension you are weak and vulnerable.

PRESS MASTERY STEP #5:
LOWER THE KETTLEBELL

When you test your press every month or two, you don't have to fight the kettlebell on the way down at all. Lower it to your chest with a relaxed arm, brace your abs, tense your glutes, and dip your knees to absorb the shock. You need to save your energy for more presses.

> *Save your energy when testing your C&P.*
> *Relax the arm and dip the knees when*
> *lowering the kettlebell to your chest.*

In training you will be doing it differently: Lower the kettlebell under control, and focus on pulling your elbow down and across your body using your lats and obliques, as in a downward elbow strike or a one-arm chin. (Eventually, once you become aware of your lat, try using it when pressing the kettlebell, a subtle advanced technique.)

Once the girya is in the rack, drop it and clean and press it again.

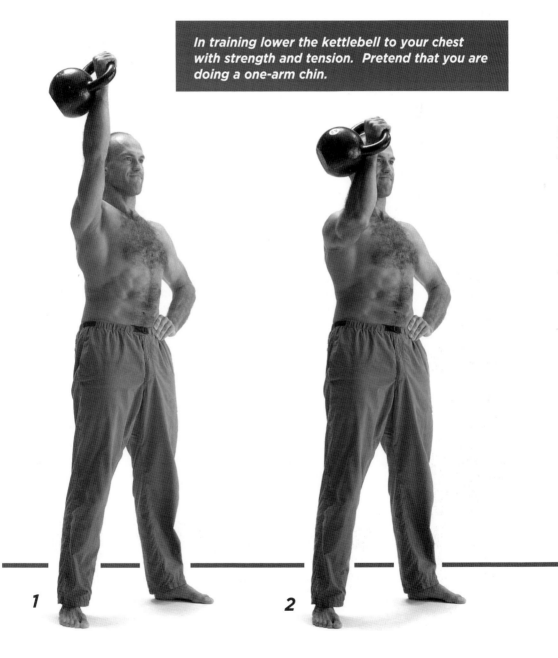

In training lower the kettlebell to your chest with strength and tension. Pretend that you are doing a one-arm chin.

1

2

There are two ways to press for reps. One is recleaning the kettlebell before each press. We call this the "clean-and-press" (C&P). The other is cleaning the kettlebell once and then pressing it multiple times from the shoulder. We call this the "military press" (MP).

The former loads more spring into your pressing muscles, helps you stay tight, and enables you to use more weight. The latter keeps the muscle under tension longer and builds more mass. In the future, once you have great technique, you may replace C&Ps with MPs on your light day. For now, clean before each press.

Iron legend Dave Draper has praised the clean-and-press with a dumbbell as "a most significant and productive exercise," and his comments apply doubly for the kettlebell: "This gutsy original exercise is regaining its popularity (trendy lifters find it tough) due to its systemic action; the entire body is involved in its execution resulting in the development of a network of muscle, practical strength, cardio-respiratory efficiency and functional skill. A golden exercise worth practicing, perfecting, and framing. Tough is good."

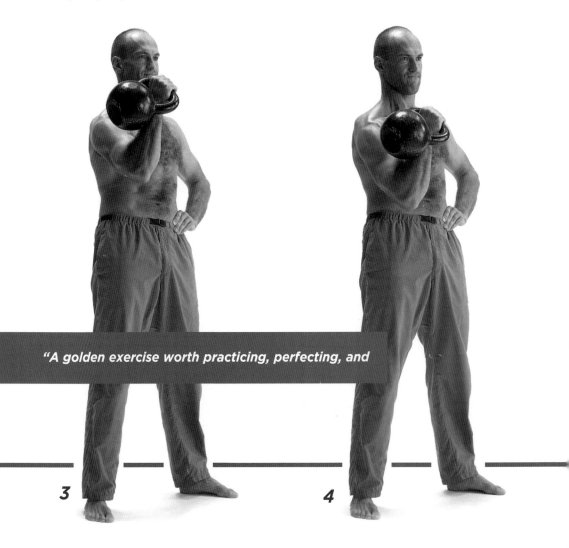

"A golden exercise worth practicing, perfecting, and

3   4

The RKC Operating System for Presses

1. ## Your press is only as good as your clean.
   a. Make the kinetic energy of the clean go straight down to your feet.
   b. Brace your full body before the impact.
   c. Store the energy of the clean like a spring.

2. ## Stay tight.
   a. Brace (don't suck in) your abs
   b. "Breathe behind the shield," while keeping your abs " braced for a punch."
   c. Cramp your glutes.
   d. Tense your quads and pull up your kneecaps.
   e. Crush the kettlebell handle.

3. ## Use solid shoulder mechanics.
   a. Keep your shoulder down.
   b. Press and lower from the lat.
   c. Don't press the kettlebell; push yourself away from it.
   d. Press in an arc rather than straight up. Push out against the body of the kettlebell with your forearm.

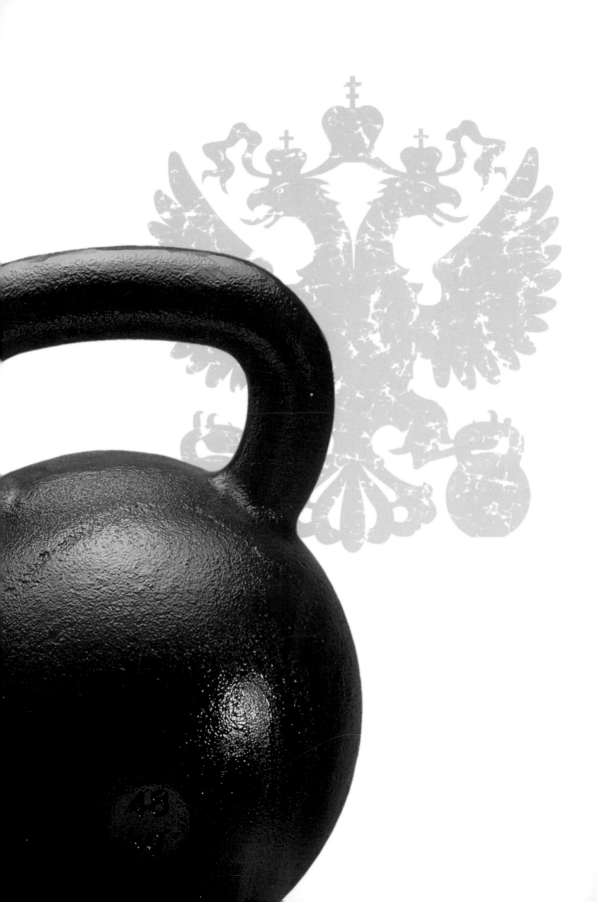

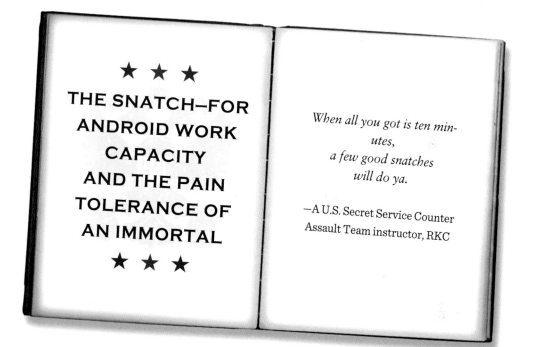

★ ★ ★

THE SNATCH–FOR ANDROID WORK CAPACITY AND THE PAIN TOLERANCE OF AN IMMORTAL

★ ★ ★

When all you got is ten minutes,
a few good snatches
will do ya.

—A U.S. Secret Service Counter Assault Team instructor, RKC

Fast and vicious, the one-arm snatch is the Tsar of kettlebell lifts. The Russian armed forces test the snatch instead of push-ups, and it is quickly catching on in elite U.S. units. You can find kettlebells in Iraq and Afghanistan, where they have deployed with Recon Marines, PJs, SEALs, and other SOF guys. The U.S. Secret Service Counter Assault Team tests total snatches with a 24 kg kettlebell in 10 minutes. The CAT operator may switch hands as many times as he wants; the sum of both arms is the total. 200 gets respect and the record is in the high 200s.

The snatch forges iron backs, hips, and fingers; develops outstanding cardio-respiratory endurance; and has a tremendous carryover to running, jumping, rucking, fighting, and myriad other physical endeavors. Last but not least, the high-rep kettlebell snatch builds willpower and pain tolerance. Bill Fox, RKC, has suggested that within a couple of years this test will find its way into the NFL. A whole lot more telling than repping out on the bench press.

TASK: KETTLEBELL SNATCH

Condition:

Snatch a kettlebell for repetitions with one arm and then the other.

Standard:
1. All of the points that apply to the swing, (see pages 44-45) minus the requirement to keep a straight arm.
2. Pick up the kettlebell, swing it back between your legs, and snatch it overhead in one uninterrupted motion to a straight-arm lockout.

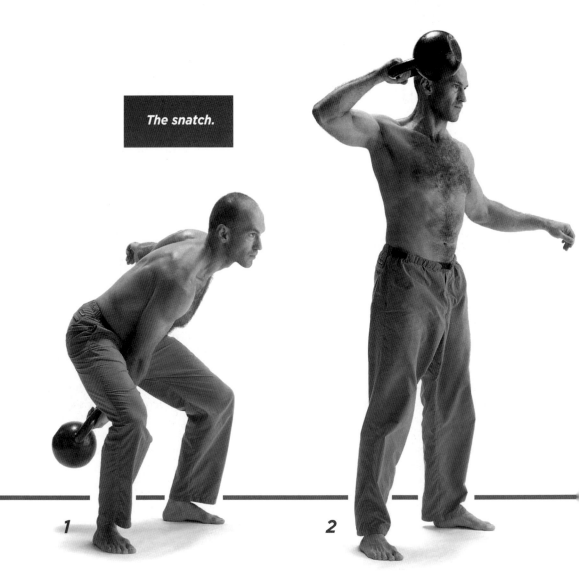

The snatch.

1

2

3. Catch the kettlebell softly without banging your forearm or jarring your elbow and shoulder.
4. At the lockout, the arm must be level with the head or behind the head.
5. Maintain the fixation for a second with the arm and legs straight and the feet and body stationary.
6. Lower the kettlebell between your legs in one loose, uninterrupted motion without touching the chest or the shoulder, and snatch again.

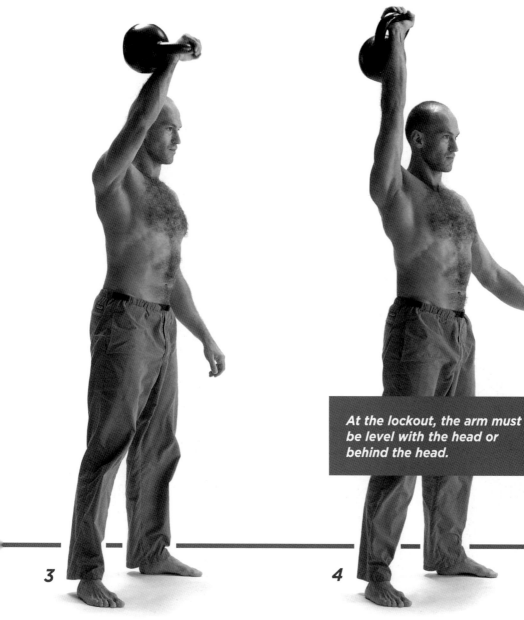

At the lockout, the arm must be level with the head or behind the head.

3

4

SNATCH MASTERY STEP #1: THE HIGH PULL

Anthony Diluglio, RKC, has significantly accelerated the time it takes to teach a victim the kettlebell snatch by introducing the high pull as an intermediate drill.

Swing the kettlebell back between your legs as if you are about swing or clean it. Drive the hips through, and yank your elbow back above your shoulder. Use your upper back rather than your biceps. Visualize an elbow strike, not a curl. Powerfully synchronize the hip and back action.

On the top of the pull, the kettlebell should form an extension of your forearm rather than droop or flip up. The whole works are parallel to the deck.

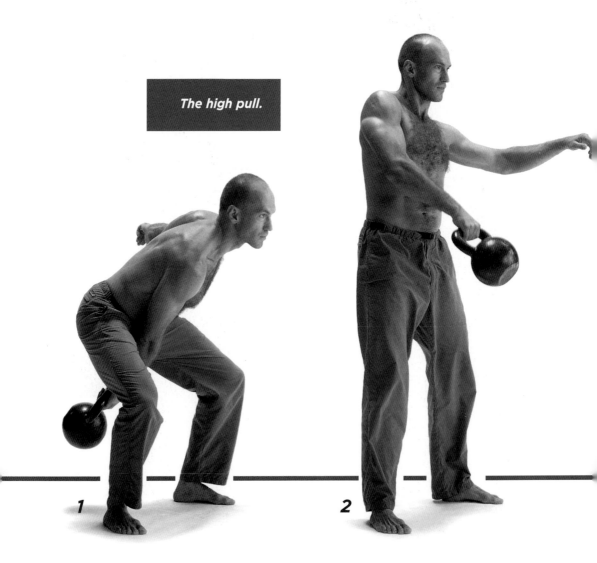

The high pull.

1

2

Aggressively lean into the kettlebell the moment you are finishing the pull, drive your hips through, meet the kettlebell halfway. You will get a more powerful upper back contraction, you will be better balanced, and you will learn another important snatch subtlety.

Aim for making the kettlebell weightless momentarily; if you wanted to, you could release the handle and grab it again without missing a beat.

Hike pass the kettlebell back between your legs and carry on.

The high pull is not just a remedial drill but a powerful exercise in its own right. Your traps will be hurting units the day after.

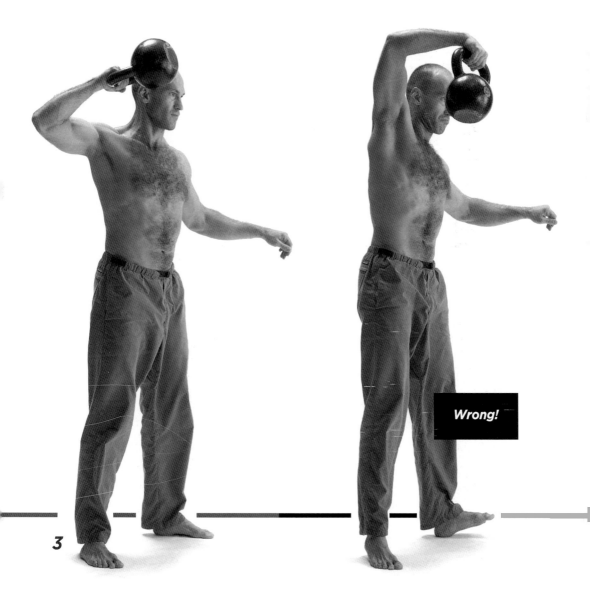

3

Wrong!

SNATCH MASTERY STEP #2: THE LOCKOUT

The snatch is powered by the hips; the arm just guides the kettlebell home. You can think of the snatch as a three-stage rocket.

The most powerful stage, the first, is the hips. They drive until the kettlebell reaches your chest level.

The second stage is the muscles of your upper back that yank your shoulder back as if you are starting a lawn mower. Remember the high pull? This stage is faster than the first but less powerful.

By the time the third stage, your arm, kicks in the kettlebell must be weightless. As with launching a spacecraft, the last stage is very fast but not at all powerful. A jab, not a cross. Your arm is not supposed to lift the kettlebell but just steer it into orbit. Quickly punch up with your fist, and the kettlebell will come home.

Remember to lean into the kettlebell. Until you are flexible enough to comfortably lean against the locked-out kettlebell, you will not be good at snatches. Work those get-ups.

SNATCH MASTERY STEP #3: DON'T BANG YOUR FOREARM

Some guys pointedly smack their forearms with the kettlebell and sport bumps and bruises on their forearms to show off how tough they are. Which reminds me of a scene from one of my favorite movies, The Magnificent Seven. It was a hit in the USSR when it came out on the big screen in 1960; my father still talks about seeing it when he was at the military academy. Curiously, it kept showing in Soviet movie theatres for decades. Would you believe they showed it to my unit in the 1980s? Consider that one movie a week was all we got for entertainment. But I digress. When one of the Mexican peasants wants to hire a scarred man to protect the village, another comments that he would rather hire the man who had left him those scars. Being able to gut out a lot of clean snatches with a heavy kettlebell is a badge of toughness. Bruised forearms are not.

Conduct a mental experiment. Swing a kettlebell all the way overhead like a torch, until it is upside down. If you keep a loose grip on the handle—as you should—the kettlebell will fall on top of the forearm. You don't want that.

Again, the secret is "taming the arc" or closing the distance between your forearm and the kettlebell as quickly as possible. **Think of the snatch as a high pull followed by a snappy punch-up.** When the kettlebell is reaching the lockout, don't allow it to spin around the handle and travel a long way to hit your forearm hard. Instead, quickly punch up with the heel of your palm so the handle outruns the kettlebell and you catch the latter softly with your forearm rather than allowing it to hit you. Punch up sooner than you think you should—at head level. Spear your hand through the handle as if putting on a glove. Spin your hand around the kettlebell rather than the other way around. You might find that the kettlebell does not go straight over your fist but rolls around your forearm. Either way is fine, as is anything in between. Develop your own style.

Don't do many snatches until you have mastered the soft catch. Practice a few every day, and get your conditioning from swings and other drills.

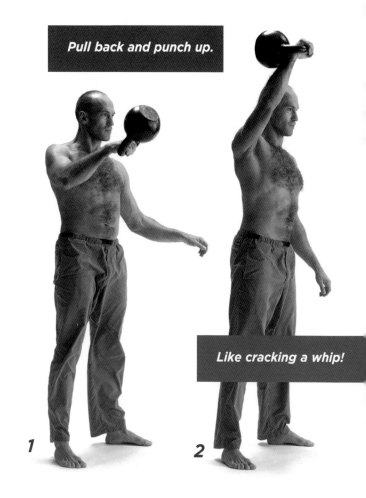

Pull back and punch up.

1

2

Like cracking a whip!

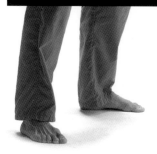

Bad news, Comrade!

SNATCH MASTERY STEP #4: DON'T STRAIN YOUR SHOULDER OR ELBOW

Not pulling with your biceps will go a long way. So will sucking your shoulder into its socket and locking the elbow the instant before the lockout. Otherwise your elbow and shoulder will get jarred every rep.

Revisit this imagery from the get-up: a "power source" in the locked elbow. It sends "energy" up the forearm and down into the shoulder. Simultaneously, the arm is "growing longer" toward the kettlebell and pressing hard into the shoulder socket. This is exactly what you should do at the moment the kettlebell is about to come in for a soft landing in the snatch.

Relax your arm once it has sunk into the shoulder. Open your fingers and even wiggle them to get some blood flowing, and down you go. Just don't let your wrist cave in.

SNATCH MASTERY STEP #5: THE DROP

The drop is no joking matter. Doing it right sets you up for another great rep; doing it wrong can get ugly for the elbow or the back.

The drop.

1

There is nothing new for you here. Hips first. Hinge and hike pass the kettlebell behind you with a straight arm. Drop it close to your body. It is too risky to practice this in front of a wall, but imagining a wall will do you good. Finish on your heels.

You may swing your free hand back sharply in sync with the falling kettlebell. If you do, swing the arm up into the "guard" position on the way up. (The same technique may be used in one-arm swings.)

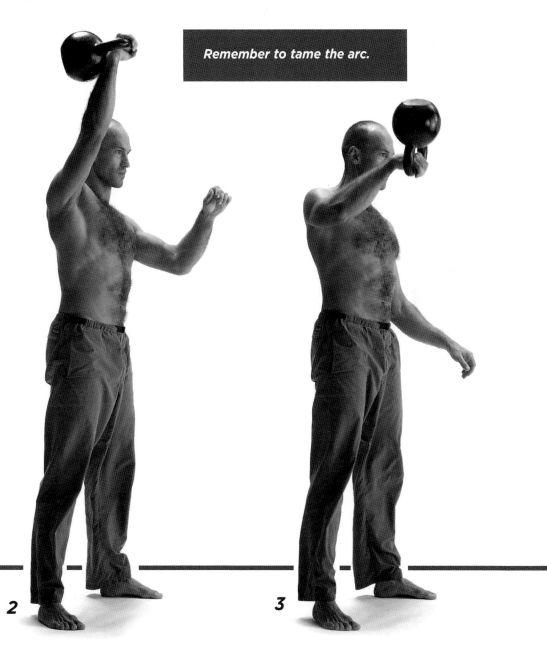

Remember to tame the arc.

2

3

THE USSS COUNTER ASSAULT TEAM 10-MINUTE SNATCH TEST

Albert Einstein once said that "everything should be made as simple as possible, but not simpler." We have come to view kettlebell training in this way. I've always loved the simplicity of the training . . . one man, one bell (sometimes two) and a field of green grass. However, while simple, I also feel that the training can be incredibly difficult, in fact, sinister would be a better description. The history of our ten-minute snatch test comes from this philosophy. We do not need incredible amounts of gear or elaborate venues, just one bell, one man and a lot of green grass.

When we developed the test, we were actually looking for something that would push the operators past their physical pain threshold while forcing them to maintain their situational awareness. In our opinion, kettlebell snatches were the perfect fit, as they tested the strength, anaerobic conditioning and intestinal fortitude that every special operator must possess. It's a well-known fact that it's most difficult to concentrate when we are extremely exhausted. Therefore, it becomes vitally important to remain focused on the small details (i.e. sink the hips, breathe through the nose, powerfully thrust the hips, stabilize the spine, stabilize the shoulder) while we are performing this test or the results could be catastrophic. We originally believed that snatches for five minutes would do the trick, but quickly realized that this wasn't going to be enough. When an operator performs this test, we find that many look fairly comfortable at the five-minute mark. It is at this point that we tell them not to worry, as they will quickly get over it. At approximately seven minutes, the looks of extreme horror begin to come over their faces and we let them know that it will only hurt up until this point, and then it really doesn't get any worse. At nine minutes, it is no longer about who's bigger or stronger, but rather about who has the most guts. At ten minutes, we have the buckets ready!

The test has been a real success and we have not had an injury to date. In addition to all operators regardless of their size using the same 24 kg kettlebell, all that is required are boots, BDU's and a stopwatch. Oh, and I almost forgot, remember to bring the bucket!

Name withheld
United States Secret Service
Counter Assault Team Instructor

The RKC Operating System for Pulls

(Swings, Cleans, High Pulls, and Snatches)

1. Hips first.

a. On the way down, crease through the hinges and pull with the hip flexors.

b. On the way up, drive your hips through without letting your knees scoop forward.

2. Tame the arc.

a. On the way down, use the "hike-pass maneuver."

b. On the way up, use the "lawn mower maneuver."

c. Snatches and high pulls only: lean into the kettlebell at the top.

d. Cleans only: pretend that you are cleaning to your waist rather than to your shoulder.

3. Power breathe.

a. Sharply breathe into your stomach through the nose on the way down, when the kettlebell is about to hit its lowest point.

b. Partially exhale with a sharp grunt on the top.

c. "Breathe behind the shield"—keep your abs braced for a punch—whenever your spine is vulnerable

4. Stay loose.

a. Keep your arm loose.

b. Hook the handle rather than gripping it.

5. Use solid shoulder mechanics (snatches only).

a. Retract the shoulder when the elbow is about to lock out.

b. Lock the elbow out completely.

A STEP-BY-STEP GUIDE TO BECOMING A MAN AMONG MEN

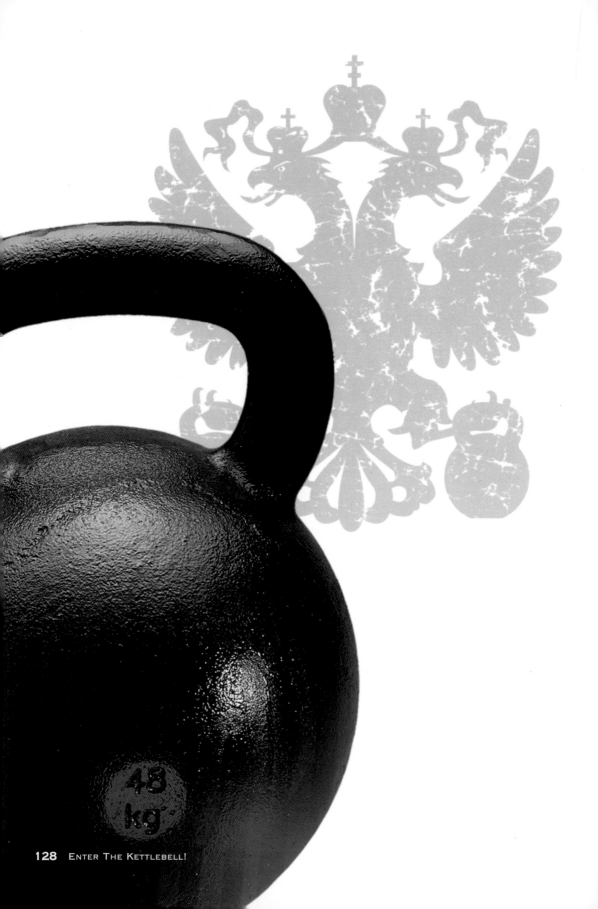

CHAPTER 4:

A Step-by-Step Guide to Becoming a Man Among Men

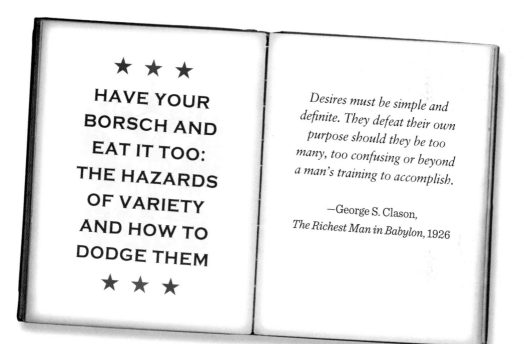

★ ★ ★

HAVE YOUR BORSCH AND EAT IT TOO: THE HAZARDS OF VARIETY AND HOW TO DODGE THEM

★ ★ ★

Desires must be simple and definite. They defeat their own purpose should they be too many, too confusing or beyond a man's training to accomplish.

—George S. Clason,
The Richest Man in Babylon, 1926

One of this book's challenges was getting a Comrade to do enough work on the basics—pulls and presses. How can one stay on a steady working-class diet of borsch when a Communist Party cafeteria buffet is available?

It is easy to start seeing the variety as an end in itself and lose focus in your training. Since telling an American to stick to plain vanilla exercises is about is realistic as ordering a kid to ignore a candy store, here is a plan that will keep your training targeted while enabling you to have fun with new exercises. Not surprisingly, it was made in the USA.

In his 1939 book *Weight Lifting*, Bob Hoffman wrote, "For the man who is really ambitious and does not indulge in hard physical work. . . a training system of five days a week will bring best results."

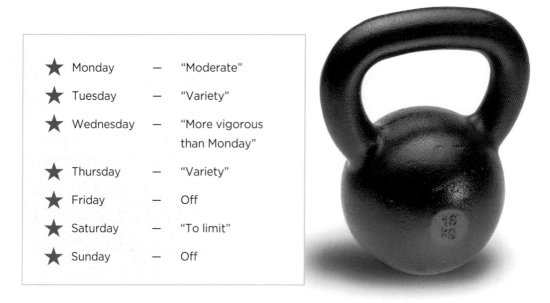

★	Monday	—	"Moderate"
★	Tuesday	—	"Variety"
★	Wednesday	—	"More vigorous than Monday"
★	Thursday	—	"Variety"
★	Friday	—	Off
★	Saturday	—	"To limit"
★	Sunday	—	Off

The above schedule for Saturday, Monday, and Wednesday is the classic heavy-light-medium system applied to the primary lifts (for you, the pull and the press). You might ask, "Why bother with easy and moderate workouts—why not go balls-to-the wall every time?"

Most complex phenomena are cyclical. Almost a century ago, bedridden accountant Ralph Nelson Elliot spent years analyzing the fluctuations of the stock market. He learned that the downsizing of the market is not a problem but a "constructive correction" that allows the market to reach a new high. The low point of a constructive correction will be followed by "an advancing wave." This is how every complex system, from Wall Street to your body, operates. Lower valleys tend to be followed by higher peaks and vice versa. That is why Russian lifters constantly "wave" their training loads. Refer to my book *Beyond Bodybuilding* if you want to learn more. For now, all you need to know is that the junk pile of iron history is littered with the bones of lifters who tried to prove the law of cycling wrong.

On Tuesday and Thursday, instructed Hoffman, "a greater variety of exercises are practiced—those that have been omitted on the real weight lifting days." Keep the intensity low on the variety days. A variety day allows you to practice—literally practice; have fun rather than get smoked—anything you like. The variety days are perfect for working on what Marty Gallagher called "in-between strength," the angles and ranges of motion not addressed by traditional pulls and presses. Do get-ups, windmills, and bent presses; juggle kettlebells—challenge yourself with any of the many moves from the DVDs produced by me and my senior instructors. As long as you stay on the ball with the scheduled pulls and presses. And as long as you keep the variety days easy. Not light, just easy.

Obviously, you can push the schedule forward as many days as you want. Weightlifting meets are held on Saturdays, which is why Bob Hoffman planned the heavy workout for this day. York Barbell grad Bill Starr had his football players go heavy, light, and medium on Mondays, Wednesdays, and Fridays, respectively. Applied to the RKC Rite of Passage program, this works as follows:

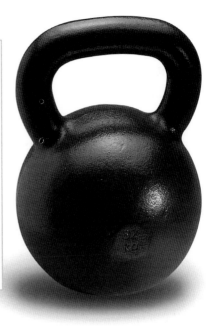

★	Monday	—	Heavy presses, pulls
★	Tuesday	—	Off
★	Wednesday	—	Light presses, pulls
★	Thursday	—	Variety
★	Friday	—	Medium presses, pulls
★	Saturday	—	Variety
★	Sunday	—	Off

You can also rearrange the schedule to make the heavy day fall on Wednesday or Thursday, the days you are at your strongest according to Russian research:

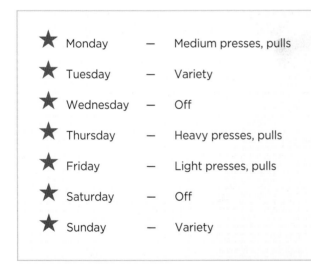

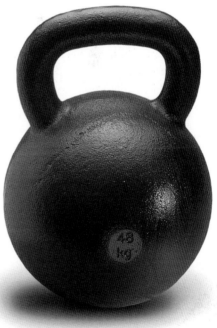

★	Monday	—	Medium presses, pulls
★	Tuesday	—	Variety
★	Wednesday	—	Off
★	Thursday	—	Heavy presses, pulls
★	Friday	—	Light presses, pulls
★	Saturday	—	Off
★	Sunday	—	Variety

Feel free to skip your variety days, but never skip a heavy, light, or medium press/pull day. Push it forward a day if circumstances force you to, but don't miss it. If you are tired, suck it up. If you have no time, skip a meal to make time. If you are traveling, bring your kettlebell with you. I know many servicemen who have taken their kettlebells with them to war, so whatever excuse you may have is lame.

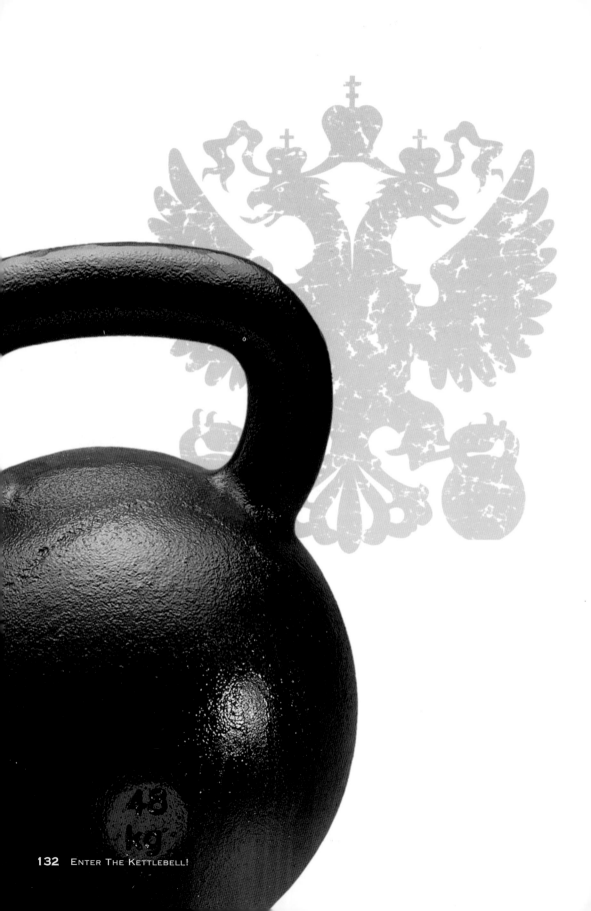

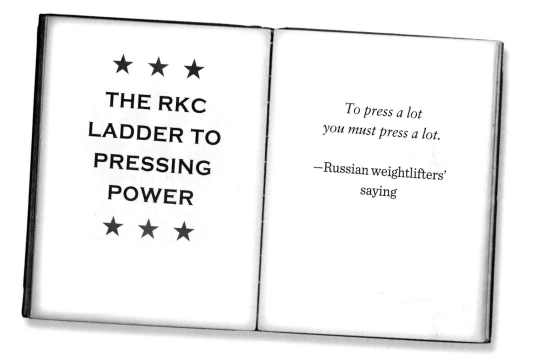

THE RKC LADDER TO PRESSING POWER

*To press a lot
you must press a lot.*

—Russian weightlifters'
saying

T he hostess at a party asks a Russian whether he will be drinking vodka or whiskey. "And tequila!" is his answer.

The bodybuilding "intensity" and "volume" camps engage in a silly, navel-contemplating argument over whether working harder or doing more work is more important. When you are seeking strength, the answer, of course, is both.

Volume is measured in kilos or pounds; it is the total weight you lift in a workout.

Intensity, depending on the event, has many benchmarks, from pounds lifted per minute to the athlete's heart rate. When the event is about brute strength, there is only one definition: intensity, quite simply, is the average weight lifted in the workout. Your call whether to measure it in kilos, pounds, *poods*, or percentages of your one-rep max. As long as it is heavy.

Effective strength building demands doing a lot of reps per workout with a heavy weight. One of the simplest ways to meet this paradoxical requirement is the technique Russians call "the ladder."

Pick a kettlebell you can clean and press—a clean before each press, that is—roughly five to eight times. C&P it once with your weaker arm, switch hands and put it up with your stronger arm. Rest. Two reps. Another short break. Three reps. Then start over at one.

Do three ladders, for a total of 18 repetitions, the first week; add a ladder the next week and a ladder the week after. Five ladders, total 30 reps. You will stay with five ladders from now on.

Although the top "rung" of each ladder, especially the last, should be tough, you must not fail! *Never train to failure!* If you want to know why, read *Power to the People!* The Party is always right.

The fourth week keep the number of ladders at five, but now try to work up to 4 reps. In the beginning you might only do one (1, 2, 3, 4) ladder and four (1, 2, 3) ladders. It is fine. Don't struggle with the top-end sets; improve without maxing out. Stay with it until you get 5 x (1, 2, 3, 4)—50 quality repetitions and almost no sweat!

You may have guessed what you are supposed to do next when you are ready: 5 x (1, 2, 3, 4, 5), or an awesome 75 repetitions with a heavy kettlebell! As before, do five ladders and patiently work up to five rungs in every one of them.

Take a couple of days off and test yourself with a heavier kettlebell. You will be impressed with your strength. Then start the process over with the heavier one.

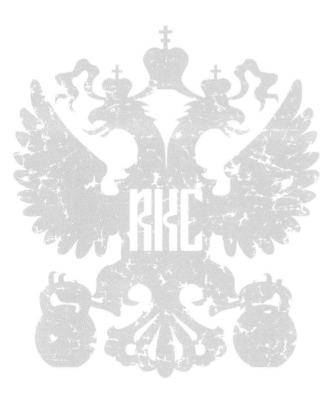

What is the Perfect Rest Interval between Sets?

If vodka is the intensity and whiskey is the volume, then tequila is the density. Density is about getting more work done in less time. It can be measured in shots—I mean pounds—per minute.

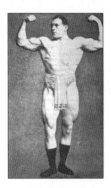

For our strength-building purposes, it makes little difference whether you have taken 15 minutes, an hour, or a whole day to do your five ladders. In 1915, *Hercules* magazine reported how Dr. Krayevskiy trained George "the Russian Lion" Hackenschmidt: "Lift weights, medium size ones, for singles for 2-3 hours twice a day, in the morning and evening, every day."

Lift heavy and stay fresh. "Grease the groove," to use *The Naked Warrior* terminology.

Building muscle is a different ball game. The complex science of muscle building can be summed up with a simple instruction: **get a pump with a heavy weight**. And that can only be done with compressed rest periods.

Either extreme of rest between sets—less than a minute on one end, and 10 minutes and more on the other—will make you strong for different reasons. Extremely short breaks will make you stronger by building muscle in the tradition of Charles Staley's EDT (edtsecrets.com). Extremely long breaks will make you stronger by improving your skill of strength in the tradition of my GTG program from *The Naked Warrior*. Medium breaks will give you a mix of muscular and neural adaptations. This is why I have not specified how long you should rest between your sets in this book. Why complicate?

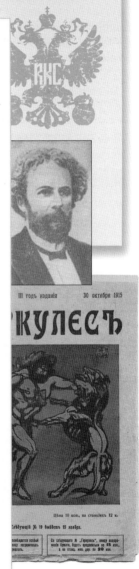

The above progression applies to your heavy day—Saturday in Hoffman's week. When it comes to presses, "to limit" refers to a hard ladder workout, when you try to top your last heavy day.

In the "moderate" or light workout on Wednesday do the same number of ladders—five, but finish two rungs below your "tallest" ladder of the heavy day. Let's say on your heavy day you did 2 x (1, 2, 3, 4, 5); 3 x (1, 2, 3, 4). So on your light day, Monday, do 5 x (1, 2, 3). You have accomplished a 50 percent reduction in volume, 30 versus 60 reps, and you don't have to work as hard because you stop at three reps instead of four or five.

On the "more vigorous than Monday" or medium day, stop one rung below the heavy day. In our example that would be 5 x (1, 2, 3, 4). You get a moderate 10-rep, or roughly 15 percent, reduction in the volume, and while it is not a walk in the park like the light day, it is not a killer like the heavy day. Medium is predictably in between.

Another example: If you are climbing (1, 2, 3) ladders on the heavy day, do 5 singles on the light day and 5 x (1, 2) on the medium day.

This heavy-light-medium ladder plan is as simple and reliable as the Kalashnikov assault rifle. Somewhat boring, but that is your problem; deal with it. Someone has made an observation that lawyers tend to be a lot more successful in strength sports than artists. Because the former can deal with the boredom of repetitive but necessary tasks. Think about it. What are you looking for in your strength program—strength or entertainment?

THE RKC RITE OF PASSAGE
PRESSES SCHEDULE AND PROGRESSION

★ Monday — Easy presses: ladders 2 rungs lower than Saturday

★ Wednesday — Moderate presses: ladders 1 rung lower than Saturday

★ Friday — Hard presses: ladders to limit

SATURDAY (HEAVY DAY)

1. Reclean the kettlebell before each press.
2. Start training with a kettlebell you can press 5–8 times, recleaning before each press.
3. Don't rush between sets and ladders.
4. Start with 3 ladders of (1, 2, 3) reps. The second week do 4 ladders; the third week do 5. Stay with 5 ladders from now on.
5. When you can do 5 x (1, 2, 3), keep the number of ladders at 5 and work up to 4 reps.
6. When you can do 5 x (1, 2, 3, 4), keep the number of ladders at 5 and work up to 5 reps.
7. When you can do 5 x (1, 2, 3, 4, 5), advance to a heavier kettlebell.

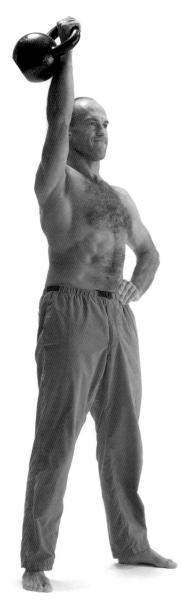

MONDAY (LIGHT DAY)

1. Reclean the kettlebell before each press in the beginning. When you have developed solid technique, do one clean and multiple military presses from the shoulder.
2. Do 5 ladders 2 rungs shorter than on Saturday.

WEDNESDAY (MEDIUM DAY)

1. Reclean the kettlebell before each press.
2. Do 5 ladders 1 rung shorter than on Saturday.

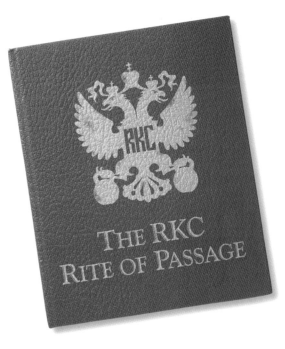

Pull-ups— a Great Addition to Your Presses

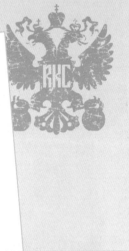

You will make even greater gains in your upper-body strength by adding pull-ups to your routine.

Use the same sets and reps that you use for your presses and alternate sets of presses and pull-ups: press left, press right, pull up, press left twice, press right twice, pull up twice, press left three times, press right three times, pull up three times, etc. If you are not strong enough to do that many pull-ups yet, stick with the same number of ladders but use fewer rungs for your pull-ups. For instance, you might do 5 x (1, 2, 3, 4) presses and only 5 x (1, 2) pull-ups. On the other hand, if you can do 10 consecutive body-weight pull-ups, weigh yourself down to 5-8RM. If you don't have a special belt to hang a weight on, hang a kettlebell on your foot, Russian spec ops style, and you are in business.

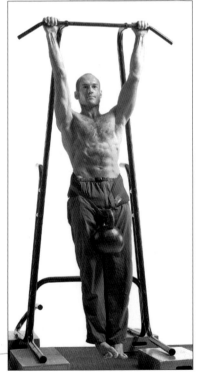

Use a bar tall enough to enable you to hang with your body and legs stretched out. Always start from a dead hang and pull high enough to touch your neck or upper chest to the bar. Control the descent and go all the way down until your elbows are straight. Pause before the next rep. Don't swing or kip. Anything less did not count as a pull-up in my unit.

You may change the type of pull-up you are doing every time or once in a while: overhand pull-ups, overhand thumbless tactical pull-ups, underhand chin-ups, ring chin-ups, towel pull-ups, wide-grip pull-ups, and so on. Just remember the heavy-light-medium principle.

★ ★ ★

REST LESS, SNATCH MORE

★ ★ ★

*Controlled fatigue is a warrior-training concept. . . .
A body trained under controlled fatigue learns how to adapt to long periods of intense pressure without reaching failure.*

—Ori Hofmekler,
The Warrior Diet

Strength and conditioning don't play by the same rules. Here is your conditioning—swings and snatches—workout.

Do your high-rep kettlebell pulls on the same days as the presses, after the presses. Your workout is prescribed in minutes, like the USSS snatch test, not in reps. Take a page from Dan John's book—pick up a pair of dice and test your luck. "Snake eyes" mean 2 minutes; a pair of sixes means you, lucky dog, will be doing your snatches for 12 minutes. You get the idea.

Follow the same time-tested heavy-light-medium template. On Saturday, your heavy day, go all-out with swings. See how many perfect reps you can crank out in the time frame your pair of dice has dealt you. Do as many or as few reps per set as you wish, set the kettlebell down whenever you must, just drive hard. You are becoming a better man.

Monday is the light day. This is the snatch day. Roll the dice again, and do approximately 50–60 percent of the reps you could do if you went all-out.

Wednesday is the medium day. Swings again. At 70–80 percent of an all-out effort. Don't be pedantic about the numbers. Close enough is good enough. The key word for this workout is "moderate"—as one of my students put it, "to a comfortable stop."

Let's say on Saturday you drew 5 minutes, went all-out with swings, and did 100. On Monday your dice rolled 10. You did snatches with your pedal only halfway to the metal, 75 reps. Wednesday is the medium swing day. You rolled 5 minutes again and did 70 swings. Keep a good record. Here is how you should log these workouts:

Sw 24 kg x 100/5 min H
Sn 24 kg x 75/10 min L
Sw 24 kg x 70/5 min M

THE RKC RITE OF PASSAGE

PULLS SCHEDULE

Each pull day, roll a pair of dice to determine the length of your round, 2–12 minutes

★ Monday	—	Easy snatches: 50–60% of what you could do in the allotted time if you went all-out.
★ Wednesday	—	moderate swings: 70–80% of what you could do in the allotted time if you went all-out.
★ Friday	—	Hard swings: as many as you can do in the allotted time.

It is your call when to move up to a heavier kettlebell.

Given that the snatch is one of your goals, you might find it strange that it is practiced only once, and on the easy day to top it all off. This is done for two reasons. First, your shoulders and elbows are not conditioned to handle a lot of snatches in your first year of kettlebelling. Don't worry, easy snatches plus hard swings and presses will equal great snatch numbers on your test days. And second, the Rite of Passage program has a lot of presses so your shoulders will be smoked by the time you get to your pulls. And snatches, as you may have noticed, involve the shoulders a great deal. So not only will you be doing snatches at half effort, you will do them after the easiest press workout of the week. And if you find that even on the easy day your snatch form is deteriorating, finish the workout with high pulls.

Now for the kettlebell "rounds," a boxing term appropriately applied to kettlebells by Anthony
Diluglio, RKC.

Elite Russian gireviks train by minutes rather than sets and reps. (Don't kid yourself that you are
elite; you will be doing the same for a different reason.) Like ladders, timed sets are foolproof and
flexible. Routines that prescribe a stretch of time to pack with work—rather than a number of sets
and reps to shoot for—are naturally adaptable to different fitness levels. This is what Steve Maxwell,
Senior RKC, and Anthony Diluglio, RKC, do in their kettlebell classes. Victims of different fitness
levels can follow the same workout, no problem.

A beginner might do 50 snatches with a 16-kilogram kettlebell in five minutes and be smoked.
Senior RKC Steve Cotter, a mutant, did 110 reps with a 32-kilogram kettlebell in the same time frame
and was just as smoked: "Very intense, I got jello legs and a chest-beating heart rate."

Sometimes one workout does fit all. Besides, a timed workout gets me off the hook for specifying
your sets and reps. Here is what Steve Cotter has done: "30/30-rest, 10/10-rest, 10/10-rest, 6/4-time
up. Total 110 reps in 5:00. . . . I put the bell down for the rest. After the first set, the rest was only about
15 sec; each subsequent set a little longer. My strategy is to try to get at least 60% of the total reps 2:00
into the test. If I get to 80 total reps by 3:30-3:45, I know I can surpass 100 reps, which I consider a
baseline for my current conditioning level. For progressive sessions, I will try to up the reps at the
2:00 mark and then go by feel/focus from there. Next time, I may go 32/32 and 12/12 for the first 2
sets (giving me 88 total by 2:00), and then stick with 5-10s for the remainder."

You will find your pace through trial and error. Don't worry about hitting the perfect rhythm of
work and rest. It hardly exists, and even the best don't hit their sweet spot every time. Catherine Imes,
RKC, put up 94 reps with a 24-kilogram kettlebell in the same five minutes, a performance most men
should envy. Still, Iron Kate was not happy with herself: "20/20, 12/12, 10/10, 5/5 . . . I probably could
have squeezed out more reps on the first set, but I sprinted through it. . . . I think I finished the first set
in just about a minute. I took too much rest between the 10/10 and 5/5 set. Otherwise, I would have
broken 100. . . . Next time I will break 100."

Federal officer Jared Savik, RKC, who has put up an awesome 275 reps, keeps it simple: "just do quick sets of ten-twenty then rest every so often when needed."

If Your Spirit Is Tougher Than Your Hands

"Anyone involved in kettlebells knows that snatches tear up the hands and torn hands equal less than optimal training," explains kettlebell sport national champion Jared Savik, RKC, on our forum.

"I've found a solution that forces a little extra grip work, but still allows for 80-90% max rep range. Fingerless cloth gloves! These dandy little buggers allow the kettlebell handle to rotate and not tear up your palm calluses and allow your fingers to catch the handle for a more secure and safe snatch. They also pad the wrist just a bit. If you want to work your grip some more, but don't like oven mitts or soap, try the GI surplus green wool glove liners with full fingers. Another excellent and inexpensive tool.

"Many of the cloth gloves on the market have the little rubber traction dots. No problem, as they are generally not right/left specific. I wear mine on the wrong hands so the dots are on the back."

Don't suck wind between sets by slumping forward, hands on knees! New Zealander Robin McKenzie, the physical therapist who has saved countless backs by emphasizing back extension and warning about flexion, explains: "...after vigorously exercising, we collapse "in a heap" and slouch badly. During vigorous exercise the joints of the spine are moved rapidly in many directions.... This process causes a thorough stretching in all directions of the soft tissues surrounding the joints. In addition, the fluid gel contained in the spinal discs is loosened, and it seems that distortion or displacement can occur if, after exercise, an exercised joint is placed in an extreme posture."

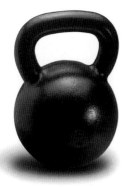

McKenzie gives an example of how just how vulnerable an athlete's warm and loose back is to slouching. A distance runner "was pain-free during the event, but was so exhausted by running hard at high altitude that, right after the race, he bent over for about two minutes, his hands on his knees. While doing this, he suddenly had severe pain in the middle of the lower back, pain that did not go away even when he resumed a normal standing posture." The runner "could not walk a step without sharp pain and . . . naturally assumed that running had caused the pain." As Rob Lawrence, Senior RKC, would say, "It's his fault."

After your pulls, do a few back bends instead of slouching. Place your hands in the small of your back, pointing your fingers downward, and keep your legs straight. Bend back slowly using your hands as the fulcrum, pause for a second, and return to the upright position. Try to bend further with each successive rep. Some shadow boxing or *Fast & Loose* relaxation exercises are also good to do during your brief breaks between sets of swings or snatches. Just don't just stand around! Slacker.

If You Have Tweaked Your Back

When you are sitting in the chiropractor's waiting room, review the safety tips in Chapter 1 and the swing section of Chapter 2. Once you are cleared to train, which could be the next day, alternate light and medium days only for the next few weeks (e.g., Monday—light, Wednesday—medium, Saturday—light, Monday—medium, etc.) until you feel confident to go all-out. And watch your form, Comrade!

Now what about the dice, randomizing the "fight" between 2 and 12 minutes? The Russian science of periodization teaches that while the athlete should stay with an exercise for a while without changing it, the workload, intensity, and volume must be varied from workout to workout. Effective training is "same but different." The exercises remain the same, but their intensity and volume are always different. "The workload must fluctuate like a sea wave: up and down, from glass calm to a storm," stresses Oleg Chelischev, a kettlebell lifting coach at a Russian military college. The dice will take care of that, from the "glass calm" of the snake eyes, to the "storm" of a pair of sixes.

Two to twelve minutes does not sound like a lot—until you try it. Note that the famous Tabata conditioning protocol—twenty seconds of intense effort alternated with ten seconds of rest eight times—is only four minutes long. "Only" four minutes long. Mind you, Comrades who have done it never say "only" again.

Enough resting now. As Jared "275 reps" Savik, RKC says, "Suck it up!"

High-Intensity Intervals— the New R^x for Heart Health

Jane Fonda called. She wants her workout back.

Wussy, long, low-intensity cardio workouts belong in the past, with leg warmers and mullets. The new prescription for a power-pump heart and great body comp is interval training, brief and intense.

"In the belief that they are building a stronger heart, many people increase the duration of exercise as they become more capable," explains cardiologist Al Sears, MD, author of **The Doctor's Heart Cure**. "Your heart already has the ultimate endurance challenge—it must beat all the time, even when you're sleeping. Instead of working longer, strive to make your heart learn to pump more blood faster and harder for a short period of time.

"As your level of fitness improves, you need to decrease the duration of your workout," insists Dr. Sears. "In other words, you cover the same distance in shorter and shorter times." After a sensible and progressive build-up, Doc recommends an interval workout that lasts only 10 minutes! It has five 30-60 second spurts followed by 1-2 minute active rest breaks. The workout starts out at the intensity level of 5 on a 1-10 scale and wraps up with a niner!

Note that the workout starts out at 5! Doc Sears is our kind of guy, who understands that life rarely affords the luxury of a warm-up: "When you are out of condition, it takes several minutes to get your breathing and heart rates up. As your physical condition improves your body gears up for exercise more easily; . . . exploit this capacity to gear up faster by increasing the challenge quicker.

"You will train your body to respond more quickly by increasing the pace of exercise sooner in each progressive workout. Don't start at full throttle, but over time, train your body to respond to the exercise load more quickly. Your body adapts to the increasing quickness of the demands of your exercise by improving the quickness of your response.

"Why do this? This is the natural state of exercise. Whether a predator or prey, in the wild creatures must be able to accelerate to 100 percent capacity in a single heartbeat. Humans have lost this ability to accelerate, somewhat recently. More to the point, this is also the very best way to be prepared for and avoid disaster from sudden increases in cardiac demand that cause heart attacks."

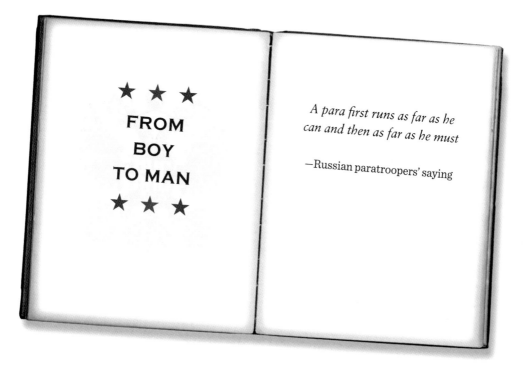

★ ★ ★

FROM

BOY

TO MAN

★ ★ ★

A para first runs as far as he can and then as far as he must

—Russian paratroopers' saying

E very month or two on a Saturday when you feel great, test yourself with the RKC Rite of Passage drills.

C&P

Loosen up with a few swings and get-ups if you wish. Test your press first. There is no point in repping out with the kettlebell you have been doing ladders with. You are training for brute strength, and doing more than five reps with a lighter kettlebell is not going to help your powerful cause. Test with the next size up kettlebell, the "heavy" one. If you have pressed it in the past, go for a C&P rep record, as long as you stay in the 1–5 rep range.

Start with a few easy singles with your "ladder kettlebell." Rest for 5 minutes, and press it for 1, 2, 3, 4, or 5 reps; then, without setting the bell down, repeat the test with your other arm. When you top five repetitions per arm, it is time to move up to this kettlebell in your weekly ladders.

If you have never pressed the next one up and have doubts that you can do it today, save it for another day. If you feel that you can absolutely, positively press the heavy one, do 2–3 loaded cleans with it for confidence, rest for five minutes, and go for it!

Kettlebell Clean & Press Rules

★ Clean the kettlebell with one hand, and pause motionless with the kettlebell racked long enough to make sure you will not be using the momentum generated by the clean for the press. Your fist must be below your chin.

★ Press with your knees locked and with a minimal back and/or side bend. The bend is difficult to judge, which is why the C&P has been eliminated from both weight lifting and kettlebell lifting competitions. You are on the honor system.

★ Your nonworking hand must be away from the body or rest on your hip. You may not push off your thigh or knee to assist your cleans.

★ Lock out your elbow completely and pause motionless.

★ Lower the kettlebell to your chest and then between your legs.
You don't have to lower the kettlebell slowly; you may drop it with minimal resistance from your arm, and you may bend your knees.

★ Without taking extra swings and without letting the kettlebell touch the ground, reclean it and continue.

★ When you have done all of your reps with one arm, switch hands when the kettlebell is down between your legs, without setting it down.

★ Chalk is allowed. No lifting belts, wrist wraps, gloves, straps, or other assistance equipment may be used.

If you have pressed the kettlebell formerly known as heavy, give yourself a cookie. Five minutes later, go from heavy to hard: the USSS snatch test.

SNATCH

Use your sense. If you are not ready to go the full 10 minutes with perfect form, pick another timeline, say 5 or 3. And if you have been swinging and snatching a 16-kilogram kettlebell, test with a 16, not a 24.

Start your kitchen timer and watch weakness leaving your body. Every rep must be perfect! Stop if you are getting sloppy! Or else.

USSS Kettlebell Snatch Rules

★ Uniform

Competitors shall be neat in their appearance and wear long pants; a tucked-in T-shirt, and military, SWAT, or hiking boots. The clothes must be clean and pressed, and the boots must be clean. The dress code will be strictly enforced.

Trouser belts, if worn, must sit low on the hips and not assist in stabilizing the spine. No lifting belts, wrist wraps, gloves, straps, or other assistance equipment may be used.

★ Use of Chalk

Competitors may use lifter's chalk to improve their grip. The equipment will be cleaned with a solution after each competitor's turn if necessary or if requested by the next competitor.

★ The One-Arm Snatch

The competitor picks up the kettlebell, swings it back between the legs, and snatches it overhead in one uninterrupted movement to a straight-arm lockout. After fixing the kettlebell in the top position, the competitor lowers it all the way down in one smooth motion. The elbow may be bent, but the kettlebell may not stop on the chest or shoulder.

The snatch may be performed with or without a knee dip at the overhead lockout. The competitor is allowed to place the free hand on the hip (but not on the thigh) and move the feet. However, the competitor must stop all movement when fixing the weight in the top position. The elbow and the knees must be straight..

(Rules continued next page)

USSS Kettlebell Snatch Rules

★ The One-Arm Snatch (cont.)

On each attempt, the judge will announce the repetition number or "no count." A repetition is not registered if the competitor failed to lock out his elbow or knees or press out the kettlebell to the finish, or if he touched the platform with a knee or free hand.

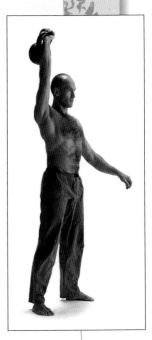

The competitor is allowed to switch hands at any time, as many times as he chooses.

The competitor is allowed multiple swings between legs when switching hands or before another snatch.

The competitor is allowed to set the kettlebell down on the platform as many times as he chooses.

Two minutes before his attempt, the competitor is called to the platform. A ten-second countdown is given—10, 9, 8, 7, 6, 5, 4, 3, 2, 1—and is followed by the "Start" command.

The competitor is allowed 10 minutes for his attempt. The referee announces every minute. After 9 minutes, he announces 30 seconds, 50 seconds, and each of the last five seconds.

A competitor is forbidden to talk during his attempt in this and other lifts.

When the competitor has quit or committed any rule violation warranting termination of the set, the judge commands "Stop" and announces the number of properly performed repetitions.

★ Special Rules and Penalties

If a competitor uses profanity or displays unsportsmanlike conduct during the execution of a set, a penalty will be assessed on that set. The penalty will be the deduction of five repetitions. For repeat violations during a competition, the competitor may be fully disqualified at the judge's discretion.

Following are three sample test days

Girevik A is doing his presses and swings with a 16-kilogram kettlebell. His shoulders are not yet stable enough to go the full 10 minutes. His test day might look like this:

Swing 16 kg x 10 per arm
Get-up 16 kg x 1, 1, 1 per arm
C&P 16 kg x 1, 1, 1 per arm
Loaded clean 24 kg x 3 per arm
C&P 24 kg x 1 left, 2 right (personal records or "PRs")
USSS snatch 16 kg x 122/5 min (PR)

Girevik B is training with a 24 and has pressed a 32 for a single. He has good shoulder flexibility, stability, and endurance.

C&P 24 kg x 1, 2, 2 per arm
Loaded clean 32 kg x 2 per arm
C&P 32 kg x 1 left, 3 right (PR)
USSS snatch 24 kg x 150 (PR)

Girevik C has already C&P'd a 32 for 5 and has been doing his ladders with it. He is working on pressing a 40 but does not think he can do it yet. So he does not bother pressing at all on this test day; he has done 190 snatches and he wants 200.

USSS snatch 24 kg x 203 (PR)

We have a man here! Girevik C will continue his quest to press a 40 and set a new goal in the Secret Service snatch, 225 reps—a number that will place him among the special operations elite.

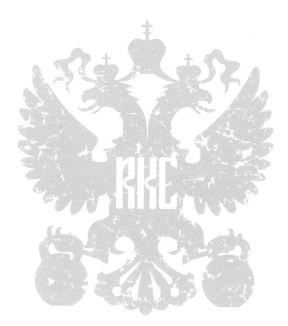

THE RKC RITE OF PASSAGE TRAINING PLAN SUMMARY

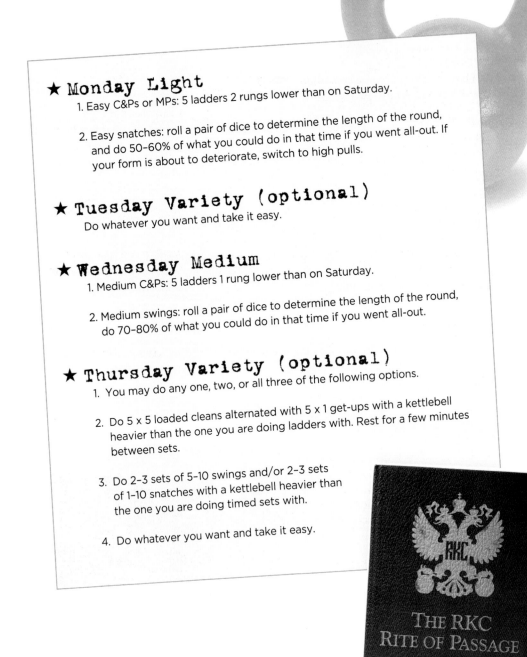

★ **Monday Light**

1. Easy C&Ps or MPs: 5 ladders 2 rungs lower than on Saturday.

2. Easy snatches: roll a pair of dice to determine the length of the round, and do 50–60% of what you could do in that time if you went all-out. If your form is about to deteriorate, switch to high pulls.

★ **Tuesday Variety (optional)**

Do whatever you want and take it easy.

★ **Wednesday Medium**

1. Medium C&Ps: 5 ladders 1 rung lower than on Saturday.

2. Medium swings: roll a pair of dice to determine the length of the round, do 70–80% of what you could do in that time if you went all-out.

★ **Thursday Variety (optional)**

1. You may do any one, two, or all three of the following options.

2. Do 5 x 5 loaded cleans alternated with 5 x 1 get-ups with a kettlebell heavier than the one you are doing ladders with. Rest for a few minutes between sets.

3. Do 2–3 sets of 5–10 swings and/or 2–3 sets of 1–10 snatches with a kettlebell heavier than the one you are doing timed sets with.

4. Do whatever you want and take it easy.

THE RKC
RITE OF PASSAGE

★ Friday Off

★ Saturday Heavy

1. Hard C&Ps: 5 ladders to limit.
   - Start training with a kettlebell you can press 5–8 times.
   - Do ladders of (1, 2, 3) reps. You are done for the day when you can't get 3 reps.
   - When you can do 5 x (1, 2, 3), keep the number of ladders at 5 and work up to 4 reps.
   - When you can do 5 x (1, 2, 3, 4), keep the number of ladders at 5 and work up to 5 reps.
   - When you can do 5 x (1, 2, 3, 4, 5), advance to a heavier kettlebell.
   - Don't rush between sets and ladders.

2. Hard swings: roll a pair of dice to determine the length of the round, and do as many swings as you can in the allotted time.
3. Every 4–8 weeks, replace the regular Saturday workout with a press and snatch test.

★ Sunday Off

With the exception of the timed sets, all the sets and reps specified are to be done with each arm.

Stay with this routine until you can one-arm press half your bodyweight and snatch a 53-pounder 200 times in 10 minutes and become a man among men. It has been said that the strength of a man's character is defined not by the intensity of his emotion but by its duration. It does not matter how hard you are training your snatches today if you quit a month down the road. And switching to another workout is quitting, period.

Straight and narrow, no fooling around. Friedrich Nietzsche would have made a strong girevik: "Formula for success, a straight line, a goal."

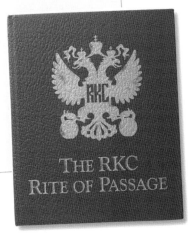

THE RKC
RITE OF PASSAGE

CHAPTER V

FAQ:
WHY THE KETTLEBELL RULES

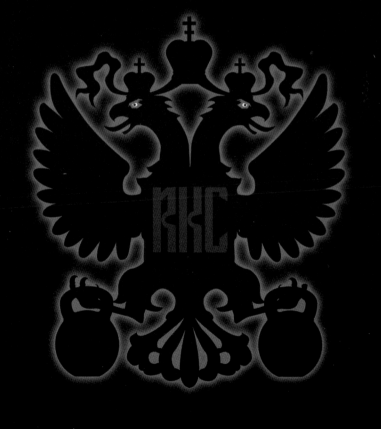

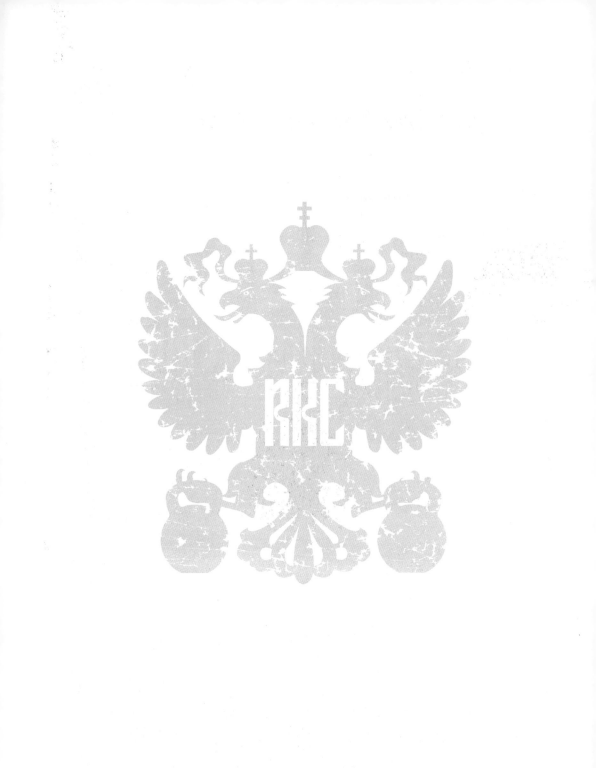

CHAPTER 5:

FAQ: Why the Kettlebell Rules

I hired a strength and conditioning coach, Joe Sarti [RKC].

I did kettlebell training for this one. I don't know if you ever did kettlebell training, but man that is some serious work...

It is all these funky, crazy body movements that you do while balancing and controlling this ball. It is very core oriented. It is very balance specific.

I can tell you, after about three weeks the density of my muscles had honestly increased by about 50%.

I gained five pounds of muscle...

I haven't gained weight for eight years. I've immediately tacked on muscle. I've never felt stronger. That was wild.

— Frank Shamrock
in an interview to mmaweekly.com
the day before he knocked out
Cesar Gracie in 21 seconds

Q. Is kettlebell training a fad?

The *girya* first appeared in a Russian dictionary in 1704 (Cherkikh, 1994).

Yes, it is a fad. I expect it to go away in the next 300 years.

Q. What makes the kettlebell superior to other weights and fitness equipment?

Some of the kettlebell exercises and their effects are unique; others can be reproduced. But nothing can beat the kettlebell's one-stop-shop efficiency.

No other piece of hardware comes close to the amount of raw power, resilience, and championship conditioning one can gain from one to two hours of weekly training with this one compact and virtually indestructible tool that can be used anywhere.

"The more I do with kettlebells, the more I think of abandoning every other form of training," writes Senior RKC Rob Lawrence. "The workouts simultaneously train *everything*. Strength, speed, endurance. . . . The thing that's surprised me most is hamstring flexibility from doing one-armed snatches. There is a great deal of truth to the axiom that all training is a matter of trade-offs, but if anything out there threatens that wisdom it's got to be KBs."

Any gun will shoot in a greenhouse, but dropped in the water or mud or subjected to Siberian temperatures, most will fail you. The Kalashnikov keeps firing. The kettlebell is the ultimate in reliability and deadly efficiency, the AK-47 of physical training hardware.

Q. Should I train with the kettlebell as a stand-alone tool or mix it up with a barbell and dumbbells?

There are two ways to train with the Russian kettlebell. One is to do it in the context of a sophisticated program that implements multiple strength tools. It is appropriate for athletes and coaches who have the education, the experience, and the hardware. The strength program developed and implemented by Ethan Reeve, RKC, at Wake Forest University is a great example of this approach.

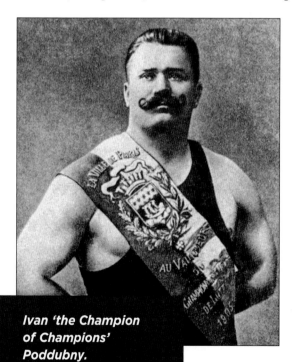

Special operators, martial artists, and other minimalists prefer to use the kettlebell as a stand-alone tool. The kettlebell can do anything a dumbbell can do at least as well, and usually better. For example, the kettlebell provides an unsurpassed military press range of motion: it does not restrict your shoulder on the bottom, and it stretches it on the top. Hang a kettlebell on your foot, Spetsnaz style, and you don't need a belt for weighted dips or pull-ups. As the Philadelphia Kettlebell Club's credo goes, "We train with kettlebells in case civilization is temporary . . . don't rely on anything you can't carry."

Ivan 'the Champion of Champions' Poddubny.

Q. How can I combine kettlebell training with *Power to the People!* and *The Naked Warrior?*

In The Russian Kettlebell Challenge I recommended alternating two-week cycles. Later I discovered that while grizzled strength coaches like Steve Baccari, RKC, were very successful with this approach, less experienced Comrades had problems. Hence two new options.

OPTION #1

Marty Gallagher told me that a perfect strength year is made up of two 12-week competition powerlifting cycles (the meet falls on week 13) and two 12-week off-seasons when a variety of exercises are practiced.

Alexey Faleev, Master of Sports and the author of a powerlifting-based fitness system popular in Russia, alternates 4–5 months of strength with 4–5 months of dynamic work.

> • Follow the RKC Rite of Passage program for 12 weeks, then do *PTP* and/or *Beyond Bodybuilding* for 12, and keep rotating.

You may GTG pistols in either or both cycles, *RKC* and *PTP*.
> • You may GTG one-arm push-ups only in the *PTP* cycle. Skip side and floor presses if you do.

When you are in the *PTP* phase, jump rope and/or do interval sprints for your conditioning.

Here is a sprint interval smoker from the record holder of the USSS snatch test: "Once per week I do a minute on, minute off workout. I will crank the treadmill up to 8.0 mph and put the incline on 12. I jump on the side rails and wait for the clock to be around 0:59 and then I hop on and run my butt off for exactly one minute. When the clock says 1:59 I jump off and walk around the room to catch my breath. After about 30 seconds I make my way back to the treadmill and stand on the side rails until the clock says 2:59 and jump back on and repeat this process eight times. It takes about 17 minutes to complete and I'm smoked. My legs are jello and I feel like puking. But believe it or not, my snatches are getting easier. I truly feel in order to get in the 250 to 280 range for ten minutes, people will need a great cardio base. Not sissy cardio, but hardcore in your face cardio to complement the KB workouts. Simply put, I run once per week for a total of 8 minutes and it has helped."

Naturally, you will have to do this at least three times a week if you are not doing your swings and snatches at the moment.

OPTION #2

- **Do PTP dead lifts on your variety days,** Tuesdays and Thursdays. Do the straight *PTP,* not the "Bear." **Skip side and floor presses.**

- **GTG pistols. Skip OAPs.**

Q. How can I incorporate *Bullet-Proof Abs* exercises into my kettlebell regimen?

An oblique-emphasis drill for 3–5 x 3–5 on the first variety day, Tuesday.

An ab-focus drill for 3–5 x 3–5 on the second variety day, Thursday.

After deadlifts if you do them.

Q. I have a bad back. Can I train with kettlebells?

Yes, with your doctor's approval.

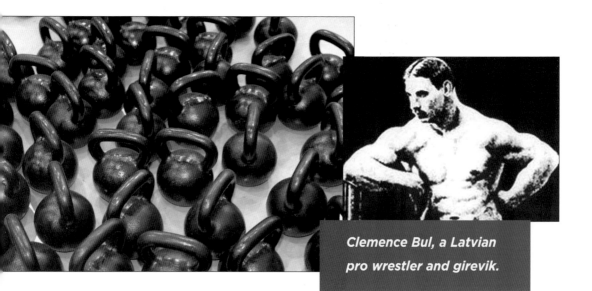

Clemence Bul, a Latvian pro wrestler and girevik.

The Top Five EXTREMELY BORING Reasons RKC Kettlebell Training Is Great for Your Back

1. Kettlebell exercises strengthen the glutes.

The late Vladimir Janda, MD, from the Czech Republic observed that people with low back dysfunction often exhibit "gluteal amnesia." And if not overcome with proper recruitment pattern practice, it is likely to lead to more back problems, since the back has to take over the lifting task of the powerful glutes. The glutes are strongly emphasized in kettlebell training.

2. Kettlebell exercises stretch the hip flexors.

In Janda's research, weak glutes were associated with tight hip flexors. The RKC system is second to none in promoting hip flexor flexibility.

3. Kettlebells develop back extensor endurance.

Professor Stuart McGill, PhD, the number-one spine biomechanist in the world, concluded that while lower-back strength surprisingly does not appear to reduce the odds of back problems, muscular endurance does (Luoto et. al, 1995). I dare you to find a better developer of the back extensors' endurance than the high-repetition kettlebell swing or snatch.

4. "Bracing" is superior to "hollowing" for spinal stability.

Misinterpreted research has lead to the currently popular recommendation to "pull your navel in toward your spine" to protect your back. Dr. McGill has demonstrated that "bracing" the abdominal wall is the superior technique. For more on this, get your copy of his breakthrough book, *Ultimate Back Fitness and Performance,* from backfitpro.com. The RKC system of kettlebell training teaches many innovative techniques to improve your bracing skill.

5. Sensible ballistic loading appears to reduce the odds of arthritis.

Repetitive ballistic loading of kettlebell swings and other quick lifts appears to be highly beneficial to your joints—provided you do not overdo it. In Supertraining, Drs. Yuri Verkhoshansky and Mel Siff state: "Joints subjected to heavy impact are relatively free of osteoarthritis in old age and those subjected to much lower loading experience a greater incidence of osteoarthritis and cartilage fibrillation . . . as one progresses up the lower extremity, from the ankle, to the knee, the hip and finally to the lumbar spine, so the extent of fibrillation increases at any given age. It appears that the cartilage of joints subjected to regular impulsive loading with relatively high contact stresses is mechanically much stiffer and better adapted to withstand the exceptional loading of running and jumping than the softer cartilage associated with low loading. Thus, joint cartilage subjected to regular repetitive loading remains healthy and copes very well with impulsive loads, whereas cartilage that is heavily loaded infrequently softens . . . the collagen network loses its cohesion and the cartilage deteriorates."

Q. What diet do you recommend?

Personally, I have been on Ori Hofmekler's *Warrior Diet* (the book is available from DragonDoor.com) for close to two years. I am very happy with it. Keep in mind that this is a personal choice, not a professional recommendation—I am not a nutrition professional.

And remember what Garfield the cat said: "Calories are meant to be consumed, not counted."

Q. Will kettlebells help my sport-specific strength?

Experience shows that a professionally developed generalized physical training program such as the RKC Rite of Passage brings about gains in athletic performance that are far superior to amateur attempts at "sport-specific" training. Because specialized training is not effective without a base of general physical preparedness. And because sport-specific strength program design is not for amateurs.

There is an expression among gireviks: "the what-the-hell effect." The WTH effect is about getting better at things you have not practiced. My students and readers powerlift heavier, hit harder, run faster, bend nails, and so on—just from lifting kettlebells. The only time they see a barbell, a nail, or running shoes is during the test! Powerlifter Donnie Thompson stopped deadlifting altogether, started kettlebelling and took his deadlift from 766 to 832 in less than a year. Steve Knapstein, RKC, ran a marathon without practicing running. No, I can't explain how such seemingly nonspecific training made this happen. But in our RKC brotherhood we don't wait for explanations to come in. If it works, we do it. If "the WTH effect" is the best explanation there is, so be it.

The amazing Russian kettlebell WTH effect notwithstanding, if you want to excel at a certain exercise, be it the deadlift or a heavy-duty gripper, you should practice it specifically in addition to your kettlebell training. To use a martial arts analogy, you will never be able to express all of your strength in a punch if you do not work with a heavy bag.

So keep practicing the skill of your sport, be it deadlifting, fighting, running, or anything else, and keep following the RKC Rite of Passage program. Once you are competing on the state level, sport-specific strength training—or "special strength" training, as Russians call it—is justified. Under an expert coach's supervision.

This is a very important point. Sport-specific training program design is the domain of professional coaches. Ethan Reeve, RKC, had no problem incorporating RKC exercises and principles into his sophisticated S&C system at Wake Forest. And I did not tell him how. Ditto for Mike Burgener, RKC, who developed a sophisticated methodology for incorporating kettlebells into weight lifters' regimens. Or Dan John, who has been throwing PRs after decades in the game. Once you become a good athlete, you need a coach such as one of these gentlemen if you are entertaining thoughts of greatness.

Burgener, RKC, who developed a sophisticated methodology for incorporating kettlebells into weight lifters' regimens. Or Dan John, who has been throwing PRs after decades in the game. Once you become a good athlete, you need a coach such as one of these gentlemen if you are entertaining thoughts of greatness.

And if you don't aspire to national and world-level competition and don't have a good coach, just stay with generalized RKC training and have a good time. Just please don't try to concoct a home-brewed "customized, sport-specific workout"!

America is on the customization kick these days. People are made to believe that personalized products are superior. They are—when they are made by a pro. But I will take a professionally made mass-market product over an amateur customization every time. Would you pick a factory-produced Harley or the Back to the Future ride your kid has "custom made" from lawn mower parts?

Q. Why are your exercise descriptions so detailed? Come on, kettlebells are not rocket science!

Powerlifting coach Louie Simmons has commented that I have reverse-engineered what top athletes do subconsciously. At the RKC we teach everyday hard Comrades how to move like the elite.

It takes a lot more instruction than "bring your fist from your shoulder to the bad guy's face" to teach one to punch like a pro. It takes a lot more instruction than "pick up the kettlebell and swing it" to teach one to swing like a pro. Anyone who tells you otherwise is either lying or does not know what he is talking about.

If you have no patience for refining the strength basics, may I suggest a Spinning class?

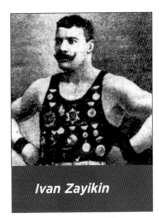

Ivan Zayikin

Q. Can I substitute the . . . with the . . .?

No. By virtue of your asking this question. If you have to ask how much it costs, you can't afford it. Once you have enough experience in the kettlebell game, you will have no problem understanding the circumstances of when you can replace the basic swing with, say, the walking swing. Or adding the windmill. Or whatever. A system is self-contained by definition. RKC is a system. Take it or leave it, but don't mess with it until you are a "black belt" in kettlebell training.

"Can I do this move instead of your move?" Tony Blauer gets irate when he gets this type of question in his close-quarter combat courses. "You can do whatever the hell you want," says Tony, "when you get back to your unit. Right now it is my system you are practicing."

Q. Once I have put up the RKC Rite of Passage numbers, where do I go next?

Get registered to vote and join the Marines; you are a man now.

RussianKettlebell.com offers a great wealth of kettlebell training information, including my books *The Russian Kettlebell Challenge* and *From Russia with Tough Love* and a number of DVDs, mine and my RKC instructors'.

There are many free resources as well: my weekly RKC blog, my newsletter, dozens of articles, and the forum. If you are not sure what your next step should be, drop by the RussianKettlebell.com forum and ask.

And if you are not afraid of pain, sign up for our three-day RKC kettlebell instructor course. It is a brutal course with a typical 20–30 percent failure rate. Rather than toot my own horn, I will send you to the website. Read what other people have to say at DragonDoor.com.

Q. If Russian stuff is so tough, why did the USSR lose the Cold War?

As I was finishing this manuscript, BBC reported, "Russian squirrel pack kills dog." As the story went, a big stray dog started barking at squirrels in a park. The rodents took no grief from the much larger predator. "They literally gutted the dog" in less than a minute.

"Man," exclaimed Phil Workman, RKC, who had sent me the link to this story, "even squirrels are bad asses over there. Explain to me again how the Communists failed?"

Keep reading the article. A local man pointed out that the forests were out of pinecones. "The little beasts are agitated because they have nothing to eat."

That answers both questions—why Russia has lost the Cold War and how it produces tough-as-nails athletes.

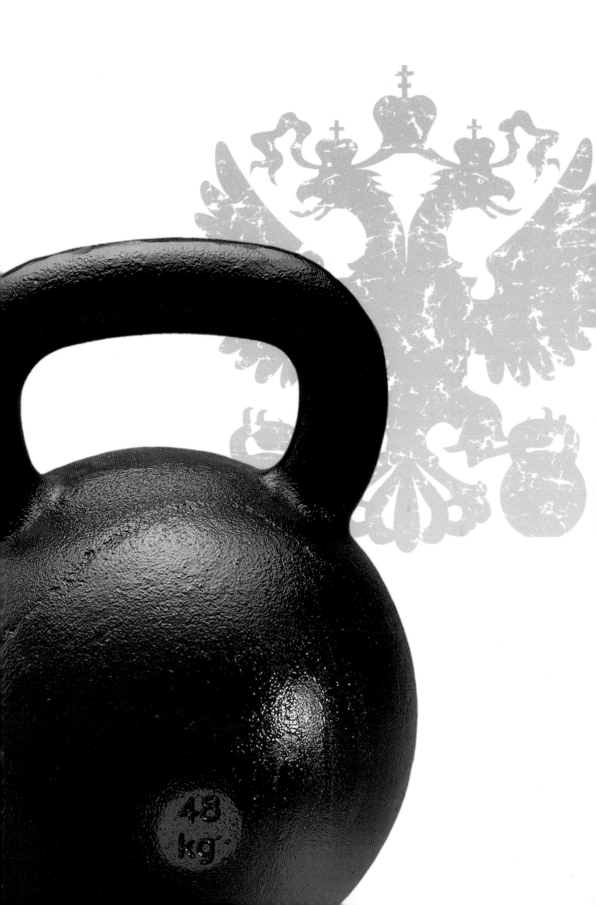

ABOUT PAVEL

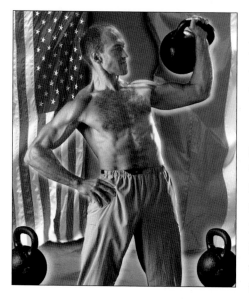

Pavel Tsatsouline, is a former Soviet Special Forces physical training instructor, currently a subject matter expert to the US Navy SEALs and the US Secret Service.

Although Pavel's expertise lies in training gun carrying professionals, his "low tech/high concept" training methods have been increasingly and successfully used by elite athletes and their coaches. Among them are UFC star Joe Lauzon, 200m sprint women's world record holder Allyson Felix, and Donnie Thompson who posted the highest powerlifting total of all time.

Pavel is the author of several bestselling strength training books, including ***Power to the People!***, ***The Naked Warrior***, and ***Enter the Kettlebell!***

In 2001 Pavel's company and Dragon Door introduced the Russian kettlebell to the West and launched RKC, the kettlebell instructor course, which became the industry's golden standard.

INDEX

F

Face-the-wall squat
  box squat and, 49. *See also* Box squat
  flexibility and, 9–12
Faleev, Alexey, 157
Flexibility, 5–18. *See also specific parts of body*
  testing of, 5–8
  techniques/methods for, 9–18, 61
Footwear (for kettlebell training), 21, 147
Fox, Bill, 115
From Russia with Tough Love, 162

G

Gallagher, Marty, 22, 157
Get-up, 61–69
  basics of, 62–63
  definition of, 39–40
  effectiveness of, 61, 71
  mastery of, 64–69
"Grinds," 78. *See also* "Slow strength" training
Grip/Gripping (of kettlebell)
  clean and, 90
  effectiveness and, 142
  injury prevention and, 32–33, 142
  types of, 32, 90
Groove, 108–110, 135. *See also* Press

H

Hackenschmidt, George, 87, 135
Halo (flexibility and), 13–14
Hand exercises/training. See also Wrist exercises/
training
  calluses and, 32–33
  grip and, 32–33, 142
  injury prevention and, 32–36, 142
Hand-to-hand clean, 26–29. See also Clean
Hand-to-hand swing, 59. See also Swing
Hatfield, Fred, 82
Heart rate
  cooling down and, 22
  overtraining and, 22
  physical condition and, 19, 22
Henkin, Josh, 65
High pull, 118–119, 125. See also Pull; Snatch
Hip exercises/training
  flexibility and, 9–12, 15–18
  injury prevention and, 23–25

snatch and, 120, 125
swing and, 46–59
Hoffman, Bob, 77, 129–130, 136
Hofmekler, Ori, 1, 91, 139, 160
Holder, Chris, 82
Hyman, Glenn, 24

I

Imes, Catherine, 3, 141
Injury prevention, 23–36. See also Safety
  for arms, 26
  for back, 24, 26, 82, 142–143, 158–159
  control and, 21, 22, 26–29, 57, 64, 110–111, 123
  for elbows, 32, 94, 122, 141
  grip and, 32–33, 142
  for hands, 32–36, 142
  for hips, 23–25
  for knees, 82–83
  for shoulders, 30–31, 105, 122, 141
  for waist, 26
  for women, 93
  for wrists, 31, 90
Intensity (of training)
  approaches to, 77–80, 144
  definition of, 133
  duration and, 144
  fitness level and, 144
  pace and, 141–142
  scheduling and, 41, 72, 73, 133–138, 139, 140, 141–142, 143, 144
  training load and, 22

J

Jeffries, Bud, 110
Jogging (in RKC Program Minimum), 72, 73
John, Dan, 20, 83, 84, 139, 161
Jones, Brett, 32, 61
Jones, Ellis, 5

K

Kettlebells
  barbell use with, 156
  control of, 21, 22, 26–29, 57, 64, 110–111, 123
  dumbbells vs., 4, 92, 156
  effectiveness of, 1, 43, 71, 81, 155–156, 160–161
  equipment used with, 2–4, 20, 146, 147, 156

T

Tabata conditioning protocol, 143. *See also* Conditioning

"Taming the arc," 26–29, 121, 125

Taras, Anatoly, 4

Thompson, Donnie, 3, 110, 160

Timed sets, 141. *See also* Scheduling, approaches to

Torso

    exercises/training for, 103, 138

Towel swing

    basics of, 51–54, 55. *See also* Swing

Training techniques/methods . *See also specific techniques/methods*

    approaches to, 77–80, 133–138, 156, 157–158, 162

    basics of, 39–42, 71–74, 77–80. *See also* RKC Program Minimum; RKC Rite of Passage

    breathing and, 53, 56–57

    conditioning and, 139–144

    diet and, 160

    equipment needed for, 2–4, 22

    intensity of. See Intensity

    load and, 22

    pace and, 141–142. *See also* Scheduling

    practicing and, 21–22, 41, 49, 72, 73, 74. *See also* Practicing

    repetitions. See Repetitions

    resources for, 162

    safety and, 19–36

    scheduling of. *See* Scheduling

    setting for, 20

    strength and, 77–80, 133–134, 160–161

    variety and, 156

Training load, 22

Troy, Stephen, 51, 53

U

Upper body, 103, 138

U.S. Secret Service (USSS) snatch, 84–85, 115, 124, 146, 147–148, 157

V

Verkhoshansky, Yuri, 105

Vertical jump (from box squat), 50. *See also* Box squat

Vlasov, Yuri, 2

Volume (of training), 133, 143

W

Waist exercises/training, 26

Warrior Diet, The, 91

Weight (of kettlebells), 2–3, 110

Weight Lifting, 129

Women

    clean for, 93

    injury prevention for, 93

    training goals for, 85

    weight of kettlebells for, 2–3

Workman, Phil, 81, 162

Wrist exercises/training, 31, 90. *See also* Arm exercises/training

Z

Zhabotinskjy, Leonid, 103

Add a Dragon Door Kettlebell to Your Arsenal—Durable, Resilient and Perfectly Designed to Give You Years of Explosive Gains in Strength, Endurance and Power

Even a man of average initial strength can immediately start using the 16kg/35lb kettlebell for two-handed swings and quickly gravitate to one-handed swings, followed by jerks, cleans and snatches. Within a few weeks you can expect to see spectacular gains in overall strength and conditioning— and for many—significant fat loss.

Dragon Door re-introduced kettlebells to the US with the uniquely designed 35lb cast iron kettlebell—and it has remained our most popular kettlebell. Why? Let Dragon Door's own satisfied customers tell the story:

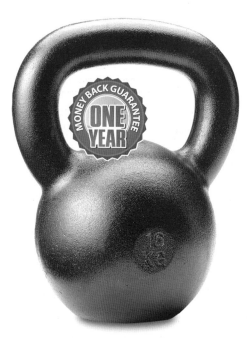

Our most popular kettlebell weighs 35lb (16kg)—and is the ideal size for most men to jumpstart their new cardio, conditioning and strength programs.

Excellent Quality

"Unlike other kettlebells I have used, Dragon Door is of far superior quality. You name it, Dragon Door has got it! Where other bells lack, Dragon Door kettlebells easily meet, if not exceed, what a bell is supposed to have in quality! Great balance, nice thick handle for grip strength, and a finish that won't destroy your hands when doing kettlebell exercises."
—BARRY ADAMSON, Frederick, MD

Continually Impressed

"Dragon Door never fails to impress with their quality service and products. I bought the 16kg last month and since adding it to my kettlebell 'arsenal', I am seeing huge improvement from the heavier weight. I have larger hands for a woman so the handle on the 16kg fits my hands perfectly and it feels great... This is my fifth month using kettlebells and I cannot imagine NOT using them. They have changed my life." —TRACY ANN Mangold, Combined Locks, WI

Dragon Door bells just feel better

"I purchased this 35lb bell for a friend, and as I was carrying it to him I was thinking of ways I could keep it for myself. Everything about this bell is superior to other brands. The finish is the perfect balance of smooth and rough. The handle is ample in both girth and width even for a 35 lb bell, and the shape/ dimensions make overhead work so much more comfortable. There is a clear and noticeable difference between Dragon Door bells and others. Now I am looking to replace my cheap bells with Dragon Door's. On a related note, my friend is thrilled with his bell."—RAPHAEL SYDNOR, Woodberry Forest, VA

Made for Heavy-Duty Use!

"These kettlebells are definitely made for heavy-duty use! They are heftier than they appear, and the centrifugal force generated while swinging single or two-handed requires correct form. I have read numerous online reviews of different companies who manufacture kettlebells, and it I have yet to read a negative review of the kettlebells sold by Dragon Door. I have both the 35 and 44 lbs KBs, and I expect to receive a 53 lbs KB from Dragon Door by next week. And as I gain in strength and proficiency, I will likely order the 72 lbs KB. If you like to be challenged physically and enjoy pushing yourself, then buy a Russian Kettlebell and start swinging!"
—MIKE DAVIS, Newman, CA

New Dragon Door Bells— Best Ever!

"Just received a new e-coat 16 yesterday. Perfect balance, perfect texturing, non-slip paint, and absolutely seamless."
—DANIEL FAZZARI, Carson City, NV

Dragon Door Kettlebells: The Real Deal!

"The differences between Dragon Door's authentic Russian kettlebell and the inferior one which I had purchased earlier at a local big box sports store are astounding! The Dragon Door design and quality are clearly superior, and your kettlebell just 'feels' right in my hand. There is absolutely no comparison (and yes, I returned the substandard hunk of iron to the big box store for a credit as soon as I received your kettlebell). I look forward to purchasing a heavier kettlebell from dragondoor.com as soon as I master the 16kg weight!"—STEPHEN WILLIAMS, Arlington, VA

Are You Serious About Your Training?—Then Insist On Dragon Door's Premium RKC Kettlebells

Since 2001...Often Imitated, Never Equaled...

RKC

4 kg	(approx. 10 lbs.) Kettlebell	#P10N	$41.75 (plus s/h)
6 kg	(approx. 14 lbs.) Kettlebell	#P10P	$54.95 (plus s/h)
8 kg	(approx. 18 lbs.) Kettlebell	#P10M	$65.95 (plus s/h)
10 kg	(approx. 22 lbs.) Kettlebell	#P10T	$71.45 (plus s/h)
12 kg	(approx. 26 lbs.) Kettlebell	#P10G	$76.95 (plus s/h)
14 kg	(approx. 31 lbs.) Kettlebell	#P10U	$87.95 (plus s/h)
16 kg	(approx. 35 lbs.) Kettlebell Narrow Handle	#P10S	$96.95 (plus s/h)
16 kg	(approx. 35 lbs.) Kettlebell	#P10A	$96.75 (plus s/h)
18 kg	(approx. 40 lbs.) Kettlebell	#P10W	$102.75 (plus s/h)
20 kg	(approx. 44 lbs.) Kettlebell	#P10H	$107.75 (plus s/h)
22 kg	(approx. 48 lbs.) Kettlebell	#P10X	$112.75 (plus s/h)
24 kg	(approx. 53 lbs.) Kettlebell	#P10B	$118.75 (plus s/h)
26 kg	(approx. 57 lbs.) Kettlebell	#P10Y	$129.99 (plus s/h)
28 kg	(approx. 62 lbs.) Kettlebell	#P10J	$142.95 (plus s/h)
30 kg	(approx. 66 lbs.) Kettlebell	#P10Z	$149.99 (plus s/h)
32 kg	(approx. 70 lbs.) Kettlebell	#P10C	$153.95 (plus s/h)
36 kg	(approx. 79 lbs.) Kettlebell	#P10Q	$179.95 (plus s/h)
40 kg	(approx. 88 lbs.) Kettlebell	#P10F	$197.95 (plus s/h)
44 kg	(approx. 97 lbs.) Kettlebell	#P10R	$241.95 (plus s/h)
48 kg	(approx. 106 lbs.) Kettlebell	#P10L	$263.95 (plus s/h)
60 kg	(approx. 132 lbs.) Kettlebell	#P10I	$329.99 (plus s/h)

US ORDERING
- Kettlebells are shipped via UPS ground service, unless otherwise requested.
- Kettlebells ranging in size from 4kg To 24kg can be shipped to P.O. boxes or military addresses via the U.S.. Postal Service, but we require physical addresses for UPS deliveries for all sizes 32kg and heavier.

Check on website or by phone for shipping charges.

ALASKA/HAWAII KETTLEBELL ORDERING
Dragon Door now ships to all 50 states, including Alaska and Hawaii, via UPS Ground. 32kg and above available for RUSH (2-day air) shipment only.

CANADIAN KETTLEBELL ORDERING
Dragon Door now accepts online, phone and mail orders for Kettlebells to Canada, using UPS Standard service. UPS Standard to Canada service is guaranteed, fully tracked ground delivery, available to every address in all of Canada's 10 provinces. Delivery time can vary between 3 to 10 business days.

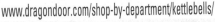

Customer Acclaim for Dragon Door's Bestselling 12kg/26lb Kettlebell

Converted Gym Rat....

"I have seen DRASTIC changes in EVERYWHERE on my body within a very short time. I have been working out religiously in the gym for the past 15 years. I have seen more change in JUST 1 month of kettlebell training. KB's build bridges to each muscle so your body flows together instead of having all of these great individual body parts. The WHOLE is GREAT, TIGHT and HARD. Just what every woman wants."
—Terri Campbell, Houston, TX

Best Kettlebells Available

"Okay, they cost a lot and, with the shipping costs, it's up there. However, the local kettlebells were far inferior in quality—do you want rough handles when you're swinging? And, if you order a cheaper product online, you won't even KNOW the quality until you have them. Dragon Door kettlebells are well formed, well-balanced and have no rough edges. Sometimes you just have to go with the best and these are the best!"
—Judy Taylor/ Denver, CO

Awesome tool for the toolbox!!!

"I took some time off from grappling to focus on strength using my new kettlebells... Needless to say my training partners knew something was up. My 'real' total body strength had increased dramatically and I had lost about 5 pounds of bodyfat weight. We are getting more!!!!"
—Jason Cavanaugh, Marietta, PA

More Fun Than a Dumbbell or Barbell

"Very satisfied. A lot of fun. Indestructable. Delivered quickly. Much more fun to use than dumbbells or barbells. Everytime I see the bells I pick them up and do something with them. Great!"—Sonny Ritscher, Los Angeles, CA

Beautiful Cast Iron

"The casting was so well done that the kettlebell doesn't look like a piece of exercise equipment."—Robert Collins, Cambridge, MA

Changing a 64 year old's life!

"After being very fit all my life with everything from Tae Kwon Do to rock climbing and mountain biking, I hit 60 ... had a heart valve repair and got horribly out of condition, It was difficult for me just to get up off the floor when I sat to put wood in the wood burning fireplace. In just 6 weeks with a 12 kilo kettlebell I've improved dramatically. The 'real life' strength that you develop is amazing. The difference to your 'core' is dramatic. Wish I'd discovered kbells years ago!"—Lowell Kile, Betchworth, United Kingdom

I Love My Kettlebell!

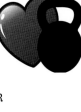

"I am really enjoying my kettlebell. When I received mine, I was so pleased with the finish and the handle. It is definitely a high quality product and when I work my strength up, I will order my next kettlebell from DragonDoor as well."—Diana Kerkis, Bentonville, AR

GREAT Piece of Equipment

"Excellent quality and finish. I'm a runner who doesn't do heavy weights; this 26 lb. KB is a great addition to my training and has made a meaningful difference, even in the first few weeks. Something about the shape INVITES you to work with it!

Highly recommended."—Matthew Cross, Stamford, CT

Maximum Results

"There is not a product around that compares to the 26 lb kettlebell. It is a health club, of its own. In my opinion anybody of any age or fitness level can achieve results. "—Jim Thoma, Shoreline, WA

The Handler

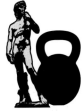

"The Kettlebell is the authority of weights. I'm 50 years old and have been working out since I was 12. I purchased the 12kg kettlebell, and at the present time used it for six different exercises. Its shape makes such a big difference; you can be creative using it to strengthen areas of your body simultaneously in one motion. In the future I will purchase the 35 kg."
—Ronald Bradley, Alpharetta, GA

Excellent Product

"I have bought two other (competitor's) kettlebells since the purchase of this product, and there's an obvious difference in quality. I am very pleased with the purchase from Dragondoor. Thanks."
—Steve Crocker, Coupeville, WA

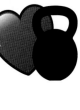

Russian Kettlebell - 12kg (26 lbs.)

Authentic Russian kettlebell, w/rust resistant e-coat #P10G $76.95